Technical Bulletin
Vol. III No. 3

I0479509

HANDBOOK ON PHILIPPINE MEDICINAL PLANTS
VOLUME II

Ludivina S. de Padua
Gregorio C. Lugod
Juan V. Pancho

/

Published by the Documentation and Information Section
Office of the Director of Research
University of the Philippines at Los Baños

College of Arts and Sciences
University of the Philippines at Los Baños
College, Laguna
First printing – November 1978
Second printing – July 1981
Third printing – March 1983
Fourth Printing, 1987

The authors wish to express their gratitude for the assistance of the following: Mrs. M. B. Quimzon, Miss C. M. Tibay, Mrs. V. E. Concio, Miss E. C. Velasco and Mr. F. Aquino.

Acknowledgments are also due to Mrs. Z. Z. Cabrera and the staff of the Documentation and Information Section of the Office of the Director of Research, U.P.L.B., and the National Science Development Board (NSDB) for financing the printing of this book.

Part of this undertaking was funded by the U.P.L.B. Basic Research Project 75-9.

Contents

Introduction

HAND IN HAND with the ensurance of man's survival must come efforts geared towards the betterment of the quality of life, one of the most important components of which is the provision of adequate health care. Steps must be taken to put medical needs within the reach of each individual, one avenue by which this may be achieved being the tapping of readily available sources of drugs and their constituents.

The Philippines abounds with plants that have been known to have medicinal properties and have been used for their curative powers throughout the ages. Recently, much interest in the field of medicinal plants has started throughout the world, and many countries have already come to realize not only their potential as means of alleviating health problems but also their economic value.

In line with the objective of disseminating information and the creation of an awareness of the importance of our medicinal plants, as well as their proper utilization and conservation, preparation of the Handbook on Philippine Medicinal Plants was undertaken. Volume I, which includes fifty of the more common medicinal plants, was printed in September 1977. Like the first volume, this book is a collection of fifty more medicinal plants, with information such as the scientific name, common names, the family to which the plant belongs to, description, ecological distribution, reported medicinal value, manner of administration, and histochemical findings for each plant. Histochemical findings for the major constituents are recorded in the text as: 1 = detectable; 2 = abundant; 3 = very abundant; or simply: + = present, and − = absent. This volume also includes color reproductions of photographs of some of the plants and some photomicrographs showing characteristic histochemical reactions as added features.

The study of Philippine medicinal plants is of special interest because of our rich heritage of these plants; the continued use of these plants among a large portion of our people, mainly in the rural areas where lack of medicines is felt; and the lack of available information on these plants. Efforts being made to alleviate our public health problems are gigantic but not nearly enough to meet the needs of a rapidly growing population. Medicinal plants are crucially important if these efforts are to succeed in improving the health of mankind and thereby the quality of life.

L. S. de Padua

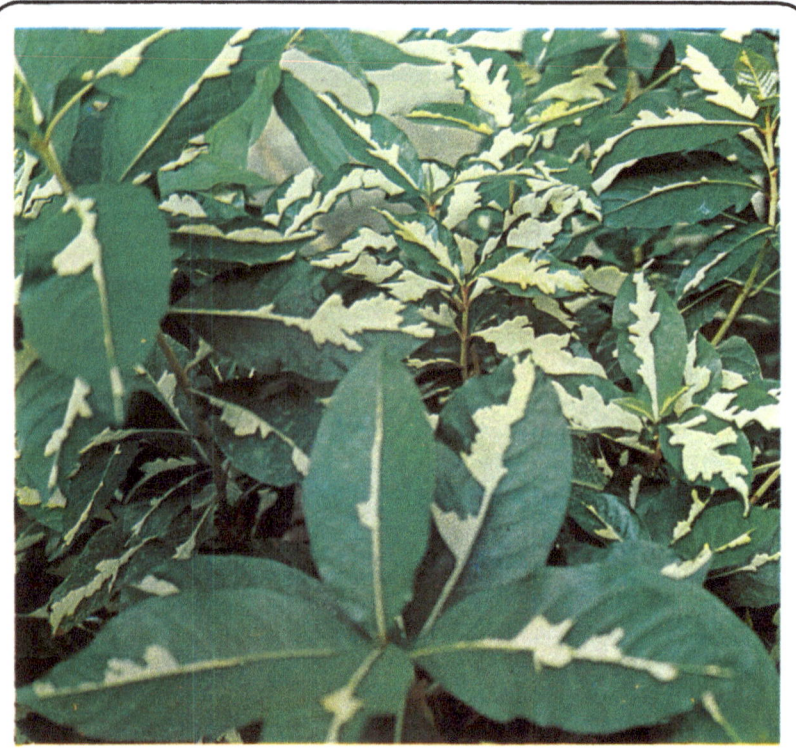

ACANTHACEAE
Graptophyllum pictum (L.) Griff.
Kalpueng, sarasa, balasbas (Tag.); *atai-atai* (Bis.); *morado* (Sp., Tag.).

An erect, branched shrub, 2 to 3.5 m high, glabrous throughout. Leaves opposite, entire, oblong to broadly elliptic, narrowed at both ends, somewhat acuminate, shortly petioled, 10 to 20 cm long, dull-purple or green and variously mottled with white or gray. Inflorescence 6 to 12 cm long. Corolla dull purple or reddish-purple, about 4 cm long.

Commonly cultivated for its ornamental foliage, throughout the Philippines; probably a native of Polynesia.

Leaf infusion is taken for constipation; also diuretic. Leaves are applied to swellings and are used as an emollient poultice on skin ulcers. The juice is squeezed into the ear for earache. Tea from flowers is taken to promote menstruation.

Fats in leaves and stems = 1 − 2; pectic substances, leaves and stems = 1 − 2; calcium oxalate in stem = 1; formic acid in leaves and stem = 1.

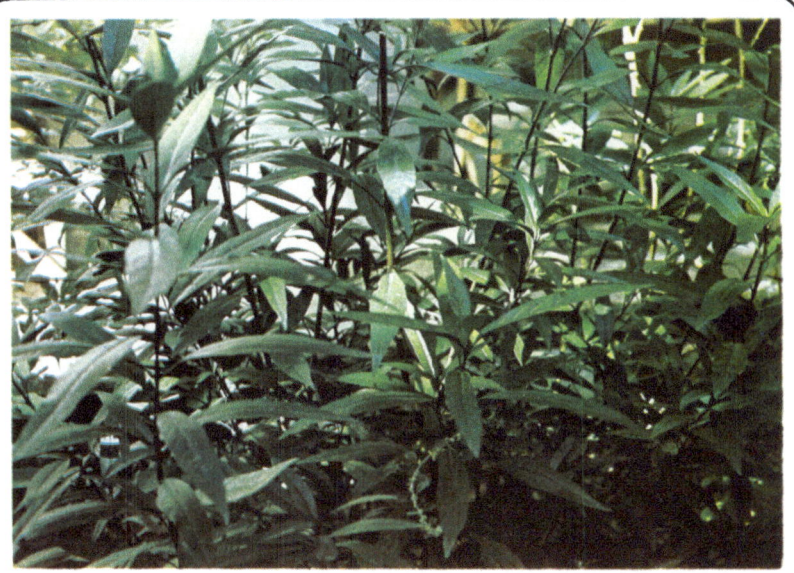

ACANTHACEAE
Gendarussa vulgaris Ness.
Kapanitulot, malabulak (Tag.); *tagpayan, kadpaayan* (Ilk.); *puli* (Bik.); *Bunlao* (Bis.).

An erect, branched, glabrous shrub, 0.8 to 1.5 m high. Leaves lanceolate, acuminate, 7 to 14 cm long. Spikes terminal and in the upper axils, 4 to 12 cm long, the flowers clustered, the lower cluster often distant. Calyx-teeth linear, about 3 mm long. Corolla 1.5 cm long, white or pink purple spots. Capsule about 12 mm long, glabrous, clavate.

Found in open waste places, hedges, etc.; widely distributed in the Philippines; indigenous.

Decoction or wine infusion of the plant is prescribed for intermittent fever. The juice of 20 to 40 leaves, extracted with water and a little wine, is emetic in coughs and asthma. The juice mixed with oil is useful in glandular swellings of the neck and throat. Leaf juice is dropped into the ear for earache. The leaves ground with white pepper is given for three days every morning for amenorrhea. The leaves and tender stalks, put in a bag together with some salt, warmed and applied externally, are useful in diseases of joints in chronic rheumatism, and in similar complaints. The root boiled in milk is given for rheumatism, dysuria, fever, jaundice and diarrhea. This drug has diuretic and diaphoretic properties as well as cooling and anodyne qualities.

Alkaloids in leaves and stem = 1; saponin in stem, = 1; calcium oxalate in leaves and stem = 1 − 2; pectic substances in leaves and stem = 1 − 2; protein in leaves and stem = 1 − 2

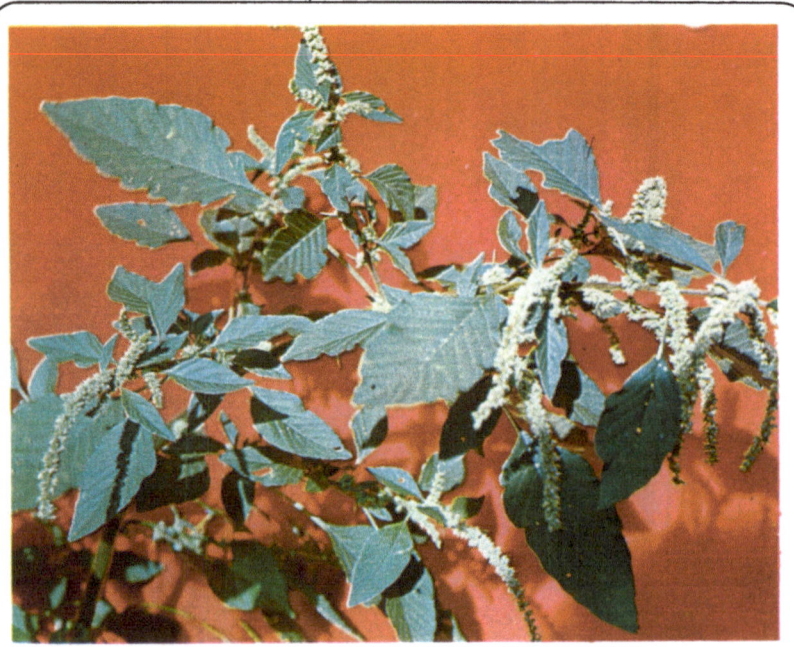

AMARANTHACEAE
Amaranthus spinosus L.

Urai, orai Tag.); *ayantoto* (Pamp.); *harum* (Bis.); *kalunai, kaunton* (Ilk.); *kilitis* (Bik.); thorny amaranth (Engl.).

A stout, erect, glabrous, branched annual, 0.4 to 1 m high, armed with slender, axillary spines. Leaves long-petioled, oblong to oblong-ovate or elliptic-lanceolate, obtuse, 4 to 10 cm long. Flowers about 1 mm long, in axillary clusters and elongated terminal and axillary, usually densely-flowered spikes, green or greenish-white, the setaceous bracts as long as or exceeding the five sepals.

Commonly found in waste places, gardens, etc.; throughout the Philippines; introduced.

Plant is used as sudorific, febrifuge, as an antidote for snake poison, as a lactagogue, as an expectorant and to relieve breathing difficulty in acute bronchitis. Leaves are considered good emollient. Bruised leaves are used locally for eczema. Root decoction is used in the treatment of gonorrhea; also an effective diuretic.

Calcium oxalate in leaves and stem $= 1 - 2$; fats in leaves and stem $= 1$; peroxidase in stem $= 1$; pectic substances in leaves and stem $= 1 - 2$; hydrocellulose in leaves $= 1 - 2$; protein in leaves $= 1 - 2$.

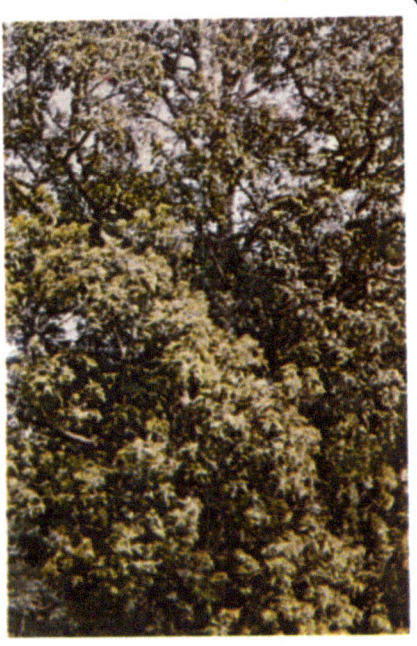

ANACARDIACEAE
Mangifera indica L.
Manga (Tag., Ilk.); *mangang-kalabaw* (Tag.); *paho* (Bis.); mango (Engl.).

A large tree, the crown dense, spreading. Leaves oblong to oblong-lanceolate, acuminate, 10 to 30 cm long. Panicles often as long as or exceeding the leaves, pubescent. Flowers yellow, small, 3 to 4 mm long. Disk 5-lobed. Perfect stamen 1, the other 4 much reduced. Ovary glabrous. Drupe yellow, fleshy, 10 to 15 cm long, oblong-ovoid, somewhat compressed. Seed large, flattened, fibrous.

Common throughout the Philippines. A native of the Indian Peninsula, Malaya, now cultivated throughout the tropics.

Tea can be made out of mango leaves to counteract catarrhs, hoarseness, cough, diseases of the bronchial tube. The concoction is used as vermifuge, for gargles, and compresses to alleviate bumps, and bruises. Leaf juice is useful in bleeding dysentery, tender leaves dried and powdered are useful in diabetes; ashes of the leaves are a popular remedy for burns. Bark is astringent and is used in hot lotions for rheumatism. Root decoction is considered diuretic. The ripe fruit is laxative. The seed is bitter and acts as a vermifuge. The dried flowers, in decoction or powder, are useful in diarrhea and dysentery. The gum resin mixed with oil is applied to scabies and other parasitic diseases of the skin.

Tannin in leaves and stems = 2 − 3; saponin in leaves and stems = 1 − 2; glycosides in leaves = 2; fats in leaves, stems = 1 − 2; sulfur in stem = 2; calcium oxalate, leaves and stems = 1; peroxidases, leaves and stems = 2.

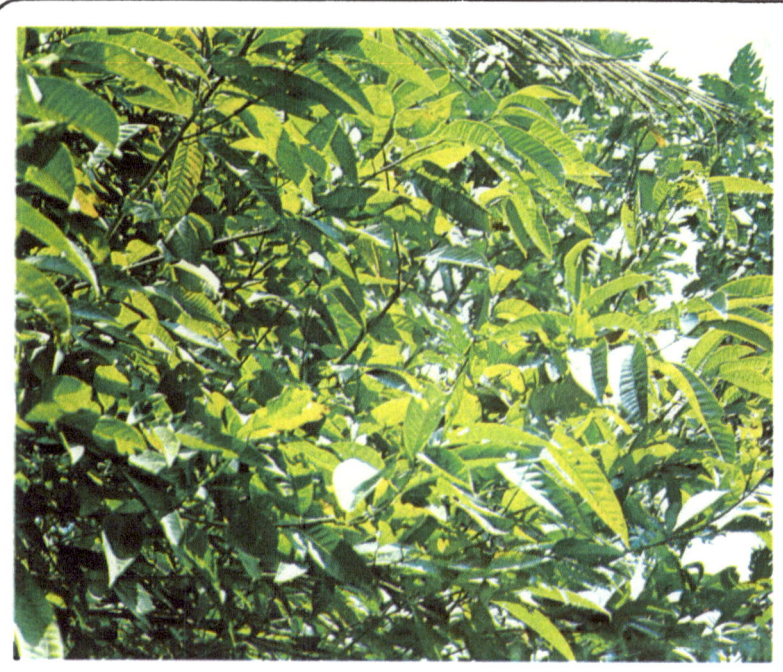

ANONACEAE
Annona reticulata L.
Anonas (most dialects); bullocks heart, custard apple (Engl.).

A tree, 10 m high or less. Leaves oblong to oblong-lanceolate, acuminate, 20 cm long or less, glabrous; petioles 1 to 1.5 cm long. Flowers greenish-yellow, fragrant, 2 to 2.5 cm long, 2 or 3 together on lateral peduncles. Fruit sub-globose or ovoid, large, fleshy, edible, with pentagonal areolae on the outside.

Extensively cultivated in the Philippines; native of tropical America.

Fresh leaves used as topicals applied to the stomach of children suffering from indigestion. Fresh leaves and fruits are anthelmintic. Green fruits and bark astringent in dysentery and diarrhea.

Alkaloids in leaves and stems = $2 - 3$; tannin in stem = 1; fats, leaves and stems = 1; formic acid in leaves and stems = $1 - 2$; peroxidases in stem = 2; calcium oxalate in stem = 2.

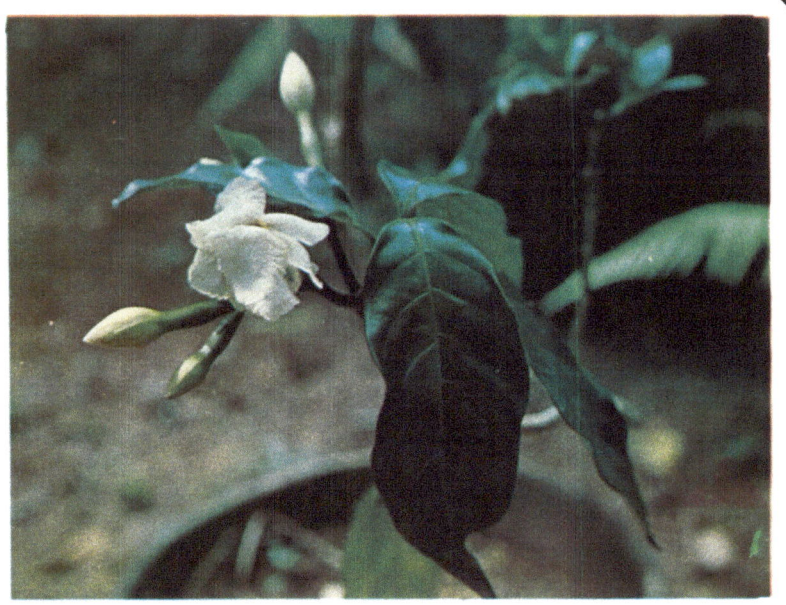

APOCYNACEAE
Ervatamia divaricata (L.) Burk.
Pandakaking-tsina (Tag.); *rosa de hielo* (Sp.); wax-flower plant, east Indian rose-bay, Ceylon jasmine (Engl.).

An erect, glabrous, much-branched shrub, 2 to 3 m high, with abundant milky sap. Leaves opposite, those of each pair unequal, glossy, elliptic-ovate to elliptic-oblong, acuminate, 6 to 15 cm long. Peduncles axillary, solitary or in pairs, short, few-flowered. Flowers usually double, white, fragrant, the corolla-tube about 2 cm long, the limb spreading, about 5 cm in diameter, the center yellow.

Occasional in cultivation.

The milky juice of the leaves is dropped into the eye to cure ophthalmia; also a cooling application to irritable surfaces, and relieves wounds by preventing inflammations, and as a decoction is given for coughs. The root is anthelmintic and a local anodyne; the root-bark is chewed for the relief of toothache, rubbed with water into a thin paste, acts as a vermicide; mixed with lime-juice is applied to remove opacities of the cornea and other eye-diseases. The juice of the flowers mixed with oil is used to relieve the burning sensation of sore eyes and is also used in skin diseases.

Alkaloid in leaves and stems = 1 − 2; fats in leaves and stems = 2 − 3; calcium oxalate, leaves and stems = 1 − 2; formic acid in leaves and stems ∷ 2; pectic substances, leaves and stems = 1 − 2; peroxidase in leaves and stems = 1 − 2.

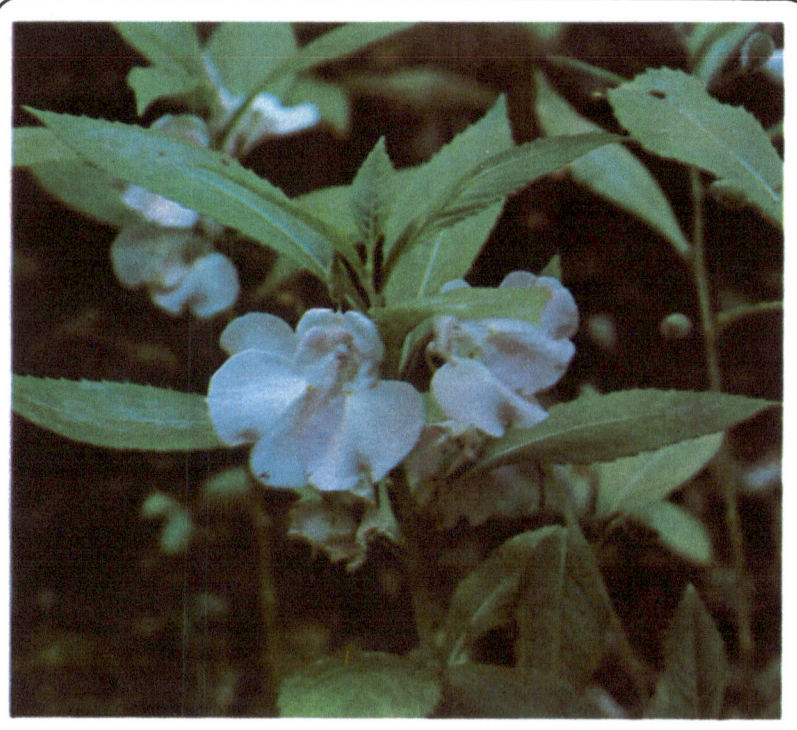

BALSAMINACEAE
Impatiens balsamina L.
Camantigui (Tag.); *balsamina* (Sp.); *solonga* (Bis.); *suranga* (Bik., Bis.); touch me not, balsam (Engl.).

An erect, succulent, branched herb, 1 m high or less. Leaves glabrous or somewhat pubescent, 2 to 5 cm long, narrowly lanceolate, or oblanceolate, acuminate, deeply serrate, alternate; petioles glandular. Flowers axillary, showy, 2 to 3 cm long, usually pink, but forms with white, red, purple, and variegated petals found in cultivation, the spur long, slender. Fruit pubescent.

A common garden plant, cultivated for ornamental purposes.

Plant decoction is used for painful inflammation, carbuncles, and dysmenorrhea. For external use on any bruise or painful area, crush fresh plant and poultice the affected parts of the body. Powdered seeds are prescribed for difficult labor. The flowers are mucilaginous and cooling and are used for snake bite, lumbago and neuralgia.

Fats from leaves and roots = 1 − 2; sulfur in leaves = 2; pectic substances, leaves stems and roots = 1; peroxidase in roots = 2.

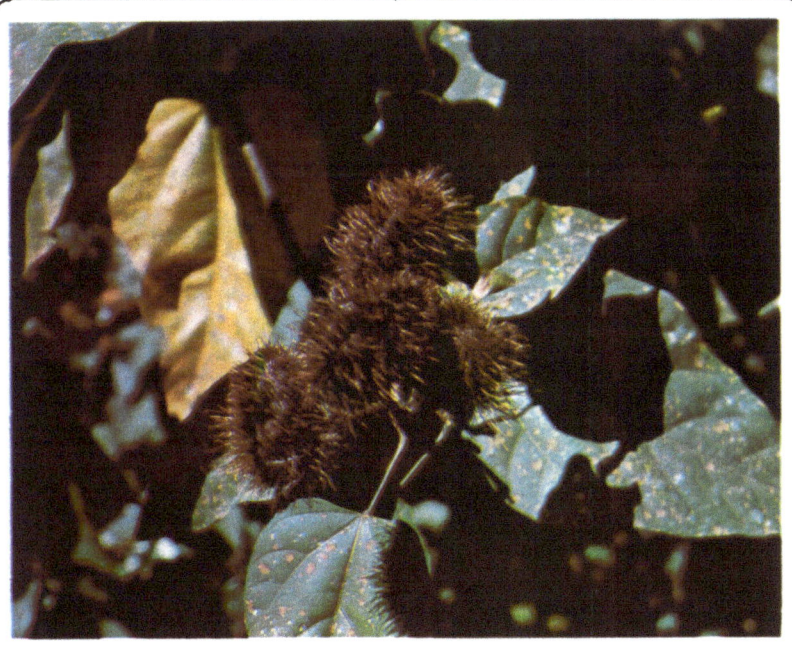

BIXACEAE
Bixa orellana Linn.
Achuete (Tag., Sp.); *asuite* (Ilk.); *sotis* (Bis.); *achote, asuti* (Tag.); Annatto (Engl.).

A tree, 4 to 6 m high. Leaves ovate, entire, 8 to 20 cm long, 5 to 12 cm wide, base broad, more or less cordate, apex acuminate. Flowers white to pinkish, 4 to 6 cm in diameter. Capsules ovoid or subglobose, green or reddish-purple, about 4 cm long, covered with long, slender, rather soft spines and containing many small, dark-red seeds.

Common in gardens, cultivated throughout the Philippines; native of tropical America.

Leaves febrifuge; leaf infusion is given in dysentery; pounded and macerated in water, leaves are diuretic. Bark decoction is employed in febrile catarrhs. Root-bark antiperiodic. The pulp is prescribed for stomachache. Achuete dye is much used with lime as an external application in erysipelas. Powder which cover seeds is anthelmintic. The red resinous substance of the seeds is considered an efficient remedy for certain skin diseases. Seeds are said to be an antidote to cassava and *Jatropha curcas* poisoning.

Tannin in leaves and stems = 1 – 2; saponin in stem = 2; fats, leaves and stems = 1; calcium oxalate in leaves and stems = 1 – 2; iron in stem = 1 – 2.

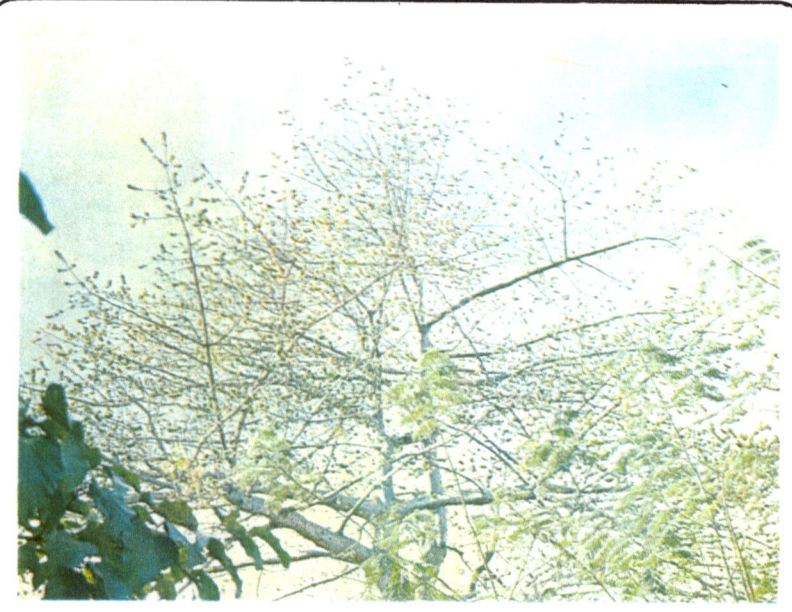

BOMBACACEAE
Ceiba pentandra (L.) Gaertn.
Bulak, buboi, balios (Tag.); *basanglai* (Ilk.); *kapok, doldol* (Bis.); *boboi, kayo* (Bik.); kapok, white silk cotton tree (Engl.).

A slender, erect tree, 15 m or less in height, the trunk cylindric with scattered large spines, the branches in distant whorls, spreading horizontally. Leaflets 5 to 8, lanceolate, acuminate, entire, 6 to 15 cm long, the petioles as long as or longer than the leaflets. Flowers numerous, whitish, about 3 cm long. Petals densely silky outside. Capsules oblong, pendulous, about 15 cm long and 5 cm thick.

Widely distributed in the Philippines, although not found truly wild; probably originating in tropical America.

An infusion, which is prepared by pounding the leaves with an onion and a little turmeric, and adding water, is given for coughs. Bark decoction has antispasmodic properties; also used in fever and diarrhea. Bark is diuretic and in sufficient quantity, produces vomiting. Young roots, powdered, form a chief ingredient in aphrodisiac medicines. The tap root of the young plant is useful in gonorrhea and dysentery. Flower decoction for constipation. Unripe fruit demulcent and astringent.

Tannin in leaves and stems = 1 − 2; fats in stem = 1; calcium oxalate in leaves and stems = 1 − 2; peroxidase, leaves and stems = 1.

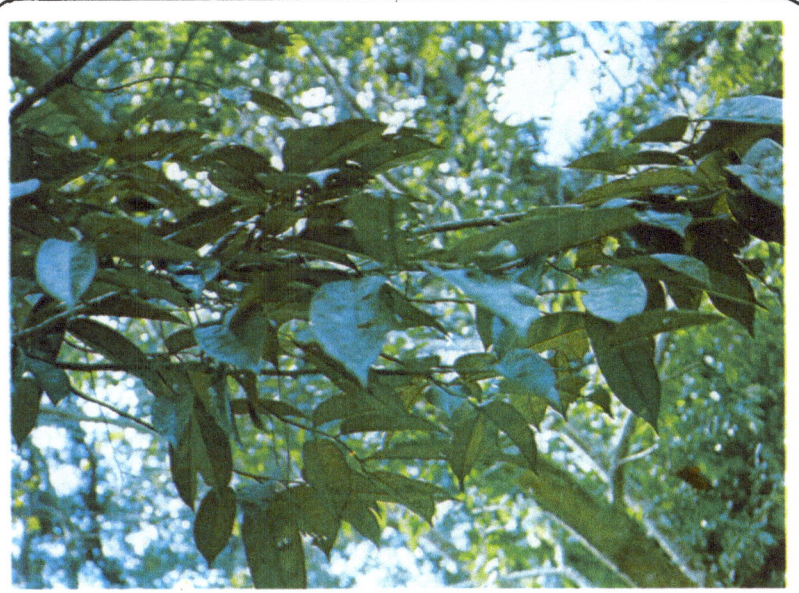

BOMBACACEAE
Durio zibethinus Murr.
Durian (most dialects)

A tree, 20 m or more in height. Leaves obovate-oblong, 15 to 25 cm long, 5 to 9 cm wide cinnamon colored, scaly beneath, and dark green, smooth, and shiny above. Whitish flowers 7.5 cm in diameter. Fruit ellipsoid or somewhat spherical, very large, being 15 to 25 cm long, and weighing as much as 3 kilos or more, covered by a hard shell with hard sharp spines. The shell breaks open into five parts to which the flesh adheres. In each section of the fruit, there are 2 to 6 very large seeds covered by flesh (aril). Flesh soft and whitish, and has somewhat the consistency of cheese and odor of very rank, bad-smelling cheese.

Cultivated for its highly prized fruit; in Agusan, Butuan, Lanao, Zamboanga, Cotabato, and Davao provinces in Mindanao and in the Sulu archipelago. It also occurs in Indo-China, Malay Peninsula, Java, Sumatra, Borneo, Celebes and the Moluccas mostly in cultivation.

Leaves are utilized in medicinal baths for jaundice. Leaves and roots are used in a compound for fevers. The fruit has depurative and vermifuge properties, and is also considered tonic. Fruit walls are used externally for skin complaints.

Tannin in leaves = 1, stem = 2 − 3; saponin in leaves and stem = 1 − 2; fats, leaves and stem = 1; calcium oxalate in stem = 1 − 2; formic acid in leaves = 1; stem = 2.

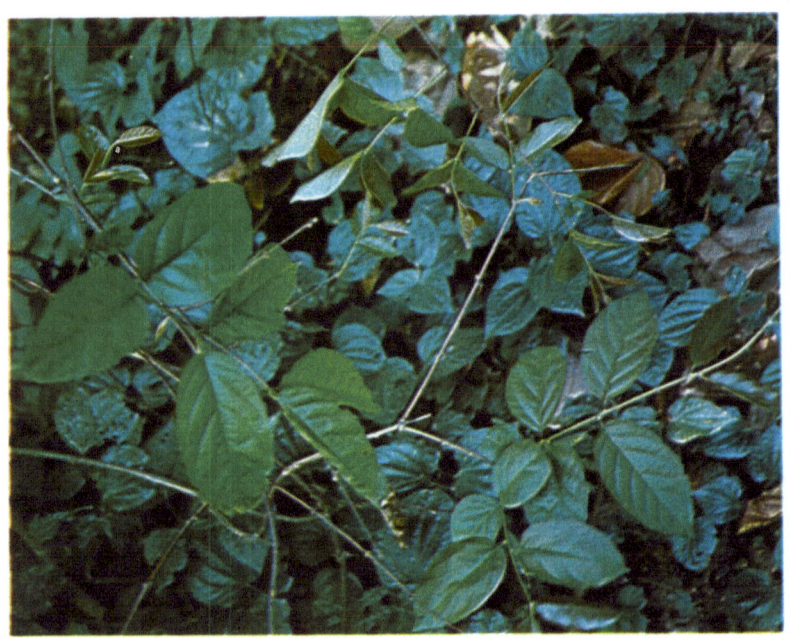

COMBRETACEAE
Quisqualis indica L.

Niogniogan, tangolan (Tag.); *balitadham* (Bis.); *kasumbal* (Bik.); *Tartarau* (Ilk.); chinese honeysuckle, liane-vermifuge (Engl.).

A scandent shrub or vine reaching a length of from 2 to 15 m when viny, the younger parts rusty-pubescent. Leaves oblong to elliptic, 7 to 15 cm long, acute or slightly acuminate, base rounded. Spikes shorter than the leaves, many-flowered, the bracts ovate to lanceolate, persistent, 8 to 14 mm long. Flowers fragrant, white to pink or reddish-purple. Calyx-tube very slender, produced above the ovary from 4 to 7 cm, the lobes 5, short, acute. Petals oblong, obtuse, 10 to 15 cm long. Fruit narrowly ellipsoid, 2.5 to 3 cm long, sharply longitudinally 5-angled or 5 winged.

Common and widely distributed in the Philippines.

The plant is used as a cough cure; leaves applied to the head in cases of headache; leaves and fruits are reputed to be anthelmintic (4-5 seeds dose) and useful for nephritis. Ripe seeds are roasted and given in diarrhea and fever; macerated in oil, are applied to parasitic skin diseases.

Tannin in leaves and stem = $1 - 2$; saponin, leaves and stem = $1 - 2$; sulfur in leaves and stem = $1 - 2$; calcium oxalate in leaves and stem = $1 - 2$; fats in leaves and stem = 1; peroxidase in leaves and stem = $1 - 2$; protein, leaves and stem = 2.

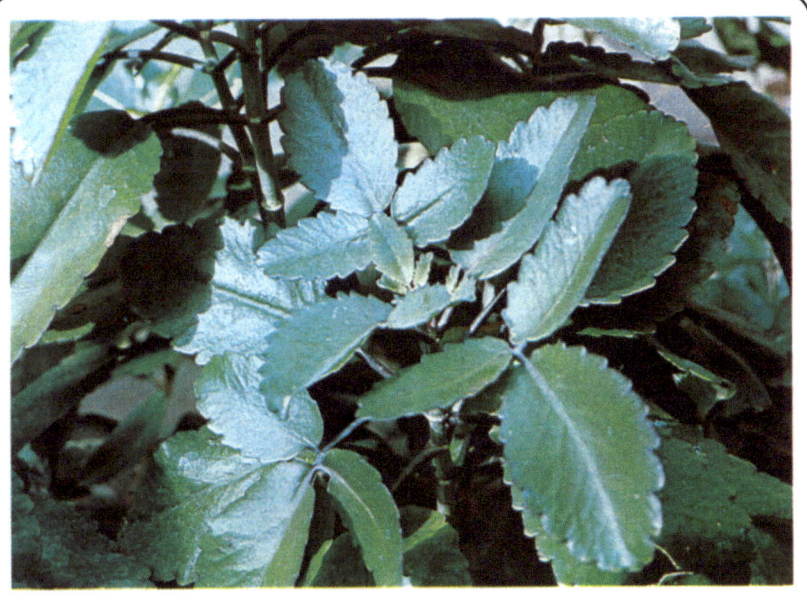

CRASSULACEAE
Kalanchoe pinnata (Lam.) Pers.
Katakataka (Tag.); *siempre viva* (Sp.); *abisrana* (Ilk.); *aritana* (Bik.); *Karitana* (Bis.).

An erect, more or less branched, glabrous, succulent herb, 0.4 to 1.4 m high. Leaves simple or pinnately compound, the leaflets elliptic, crenate. usually about 10 cm long, thick and succulent. Flowers paniculate, pendulous. Calyx brownish or purplish, 3.5 to 4 cm long, cylindric. Corolla about 5 cm long inflated at the base, then constricted, the exerted parts reddish or purplish, the lobes acuminate.

Common in thickets and open places, widely distributed in the Philippines.

Pounded leaves mixed with small amount of salt is applied to the lower part of the abdomen to relieve the patient suffering from dysuria. Leaves are used as an astringent, and antiseptic and as counterirritant against poisonous insect bites. The fresh leaves, pounded, are also applied to sprains, and burns, and as poultices on eczema, and boils and other skin infection; the juice mixed with lard is used in diarrhea, dysentery, cholera, phthisis; for earache and opthalmia; heated over a fire, are applied to wounds and bruises; also as an emollient and refrigerant over a face swollen because of neuralgia or tooth trouble.

Tannin in leaves and stems = 1 − 2; peroxidase in stem = 1; calcium oxalate, leaves and stem = 1 − 2; sulfur in leaves and stem = 1; formic acid in leaves and stem = 1 − 2.

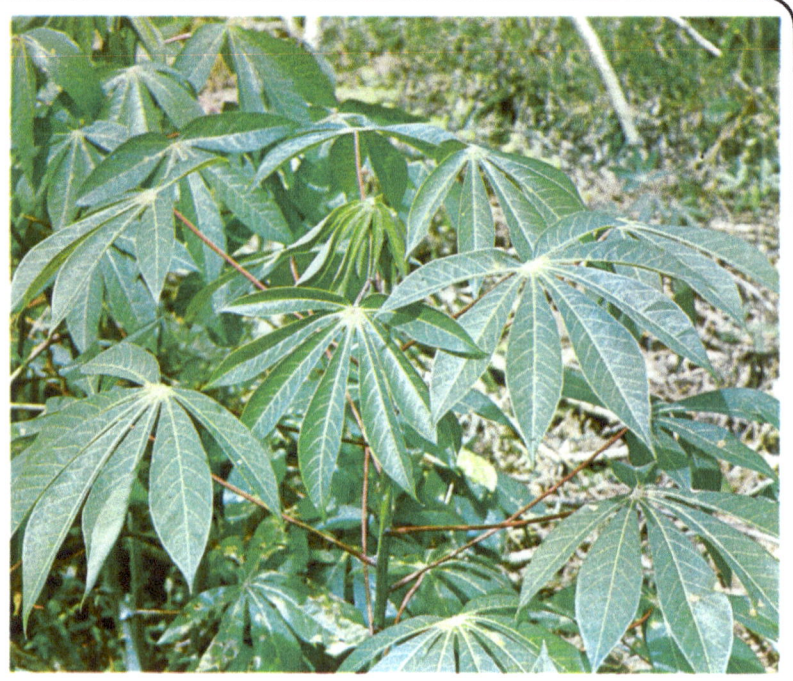

EUPHORBIACEAE
Manihot esculenta Crantz
Kamoteng-kahoy (Tag.); *balangai* (Bis.); *kamote ti moro* (Ilk.); cassava, Manioc, tapioca plant (Engl.).

An erect, glabrous, suffrutescent or shrubby plant, 1.5 to 3 m high from stout fleshy roots. Leaves 10 to 20 cm long, pale beneath, palmately divided nearly to the base into 3 to 7, lanceolate to oblong-lanceolate, entire, acuminate segments, some of the upper leaves often entire. Inflorescence axillary, lax, few-flowered. Flowers about 1 cm long. Capsules ovoid, about 1.5 cm long, longitudinally narrowly 6-winged.

   Widely distributed in the Philippines in cultivation; a native of tropical America.

   Pounded leaves are applied as a compress to the head in fevers and headaches. Decoction of the bark of the trunk is considered antirheumatic. Bark decoction is anthelmintic. The pounded tuber is applied to ulcerated wounds; also considered antiseptic, and is used to preserve meat. Starch from tuber is used for rash of children.

   Saponin in leaves = 2; glycosides, leaves and stem = $1 - 2$; tannin in leaves and stem = $1 - 2$; calcium oxalate in stem = 2; iron leaves and root = 1; peroxidase in stem = $1 - 2$; roots = ?.

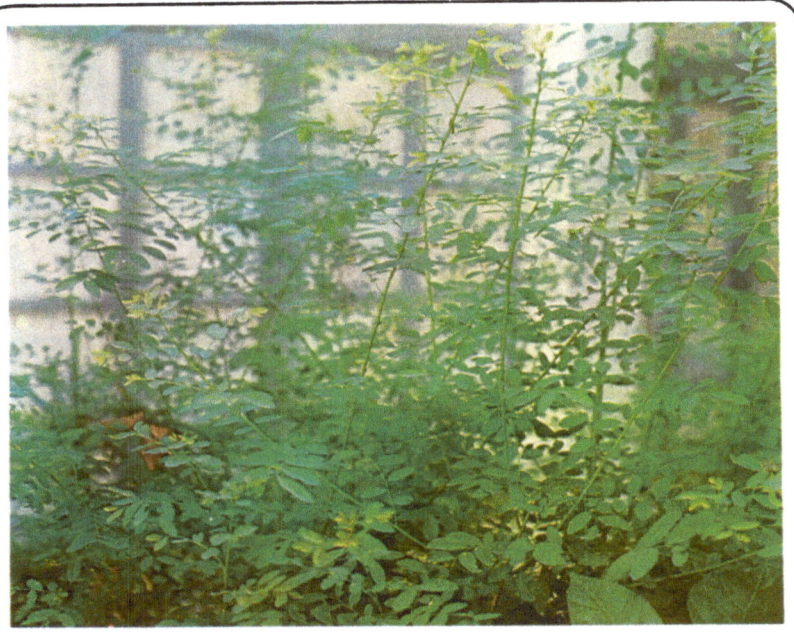

EUPHORBIACEAE
Phyllanthus reticulatus Poir.
Malatinta, tintatintahan (Tag.); *matang-bulud* (Bik.).

An erect, somewhat scandent shrub, 1.5 to 5 m high, the branches, elongated, often pendulous, somewhat pubescent or glabrous. Leaves distichous, oblong to elliptic-oblong, 1.5 to 4 cm long, obtuse or acute, rather pale beneath, short-petioled, base rounded or obtuse. Flowers axillary, solitary or few in each axil, slenderly pedicelled, 2 to 3 mm long, green tinged with purple. Fruit depressed-globose, soft and fleshy, smooth, black when mature, 5 to 7 mm in diameter.

Very common in thickets, hedges, etc.; widely distributed in the Philippines.

The leaves are employed as diuretic and the juice is used for diarrhea in infants; made into a pill with camphor, and allowed to dissolve in the mouth is a remedy for bleeding gums; powdered, is used as a local application to sores and burns. Juice from the stem, dropped into the eyes can cure sore eyes. Decoction or infusion of dried bark is diuretic, astringent and given for dysentery. Root decoction is prescribed for asthma. The fruit is astringent to the bowel and is useful in inflammations and diseases of the blood.

Saponin in leaves = 1, stem = 1 − 2; tannin in leaves = 1, stem = 1 − 2; sulfur in stem = 1; formic acid in leaves and stem = 1 − 2; peroxidase, leaves and stem = 1 − 2.

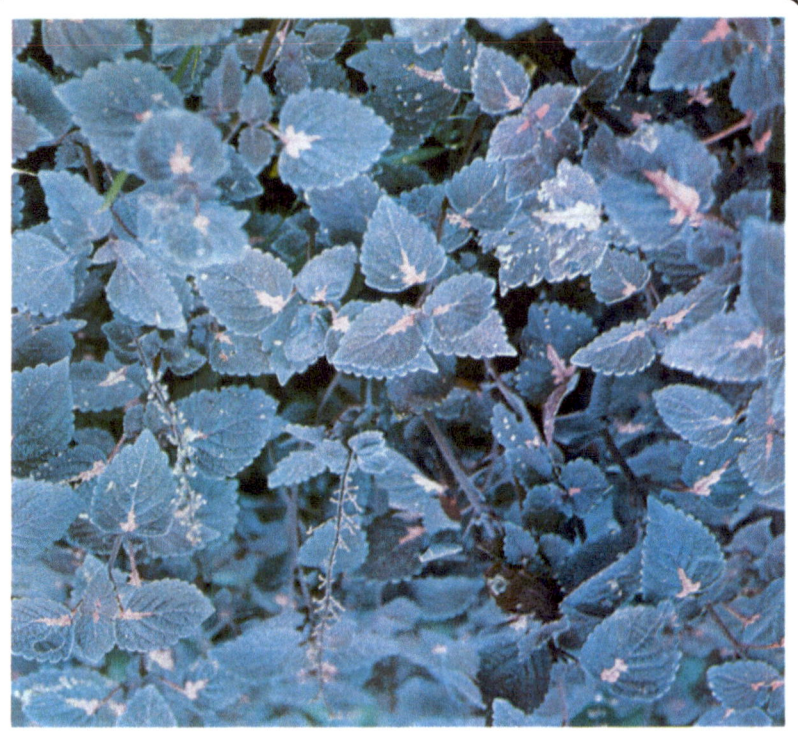

LABIATAE
Coleus scutellarioides (L.)
Mayana, maliana (Tag., Bis., Pamp.); *dapoyana* (Bis.); *lapunaya, taponaya* (Bis.).

An erect, branched, somewhat succulent, annual herb, 1 m high or less. the leaves variously colored, usually more or less pubescent. Stems usually purplish, 4-angled. Leaves ovate, rather coarsely toothed, 5 to 10 cm long. in the most common form uniformly velvety-purple. Inflorescence terminal. simple or branched, 15 to 30 cm long. Flowers purplish. numerous, in lax verticils of cymes or racemes, the pedicels about 4 mm long. Calyx green, about 2.5 mm long, the upper lip ovate, obtuse, the lateral lobes short, ovate. the lower one 2-cleft; corolla about 11 mm long.

Generally cultivated for its ornamental foliage.

Decoction of the plant taken internally is a cure for dyspepsia and also dropped into the eyes for opthalmia. Poultice for headaches and wounds.

Tannin in leaves and stem = 1; fats in leaves and stem = 1: pectic substances in leaves = 2; stem = 1; phytosterol in stem = 1; calcium oxalate in leaves and stem = 1.

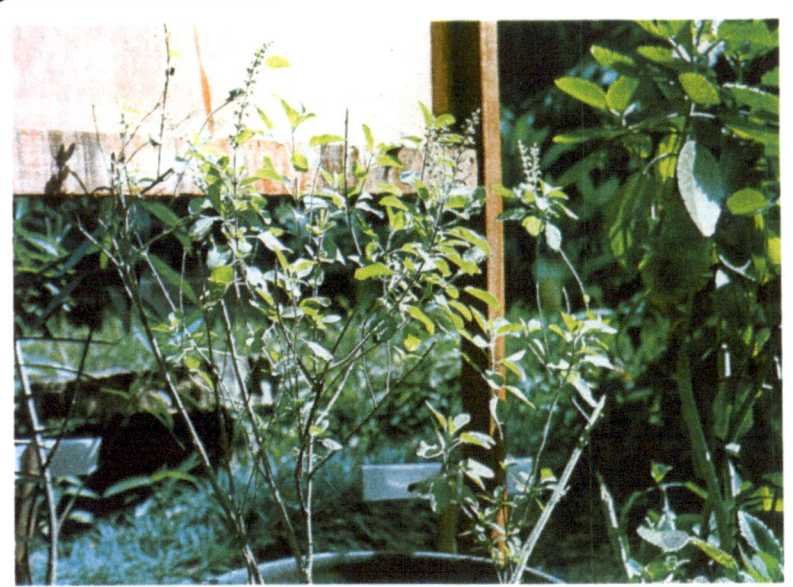

LABIATAE
Ocimum sanctum L.

Solasi, balanoi (Tag.); *albahaca* (Sp., Tag.); *colocogo, camange* (Bis.); *bidai* (Ilk.); *kamangkau* (Bik.); *loko-loko* (Pamp., Tag.); sacred basil, Holy basil (Engl.).

An erect, herbaceous or suffrutescent, branched plant, 1 m high or less, the stems and younger parts pubescent with spreading hairs. Leaves oblong-ovate, obtuse, somewhat toothed, 2 to 4.5 cm long. Racemes 5 to 14 cm long, sometimes panicled. Pedicels about as long as the calyx, spreading, curved. Calyx at time of flowering about 3 mm long, somewhat larger in fruit, the two lower teeth long-awned, the upper one broadly oblong, the lateral ones very broad, mucronate. Corolla pink or purplish, but a little longer than the calyx.

Cultivated for its very fragrant leaves; throughout the Philippines; introduced.

Dried plant in decoction remedy for catarrh, bronchitis, and diarrhea. Juice of leaves applied to the skin in ringworm and other skin diseases; dropped into the ear for earache. Decoction of leaves is used as an aromatic bath. Decoction of roots and leaves specified for gonorrhea, used as baths to relieve rheumatic pains and paralysis. Root decoction is used as a diaphoretic in malarial fever. Seed decoction demulcent.

Tannin in leaves and stem = 1; sulfur in stem = 1; fats in leaves and stem = 1 − 2; calcium oxalate, leaves and stems = 1 − 2; peroxidase in stem = 1 − 2; formic acid, leaves and stem = 1 − 2.

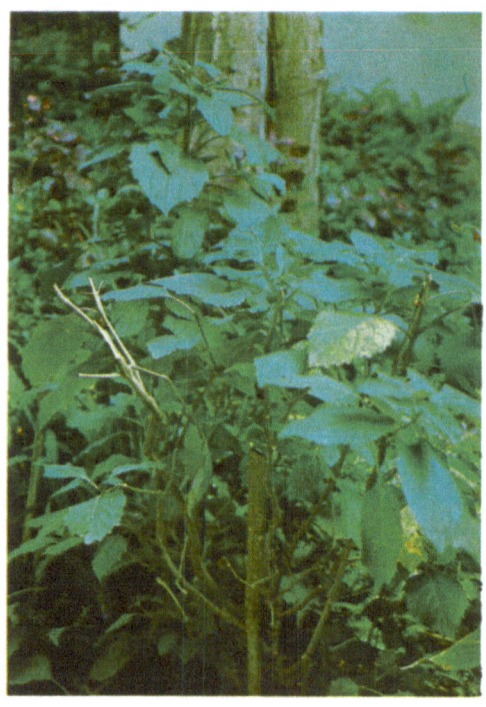

LABIATAE
Pogostemon cablin (Blanco) Benth.
Cablin, cadling, cadlom (Tag.); *kabling* (Pamp., Tag.); *kadling* (Tag., Bis.); *pacholi* (Sp.); patchouli (Engl.).

An erect, branched, pubescent herb, 0.5 to 1 m high, aromatic when crushed. Leaves ovate to oblong-ovate, acute or obtuse, 5 to 11 cm long, usually coarsely and doubly toothed or crenate. Spikes terminal and axillary, panicled, dense, sometimes interrupted, 2 to 8 cm long, 1 to 1.5 cm in diameter, pubescent. Calyx about 6 mm long. Corolla pink-purple, 8 mm long, the lobes obtuse. Bracts about as long as the calyx.

Cultivated for its fragrant leaves.

An infusion of the fresh leaves is given internally to allay painful menstruation and also as an emmenagogue; employed in baths; said to have an antirheumatic action, and is also recommended for nervous troubles. Leaves are used as an insecticide, as a repellant of cockroaches, moths, ants, including leeches. Leaves are often crushed with gogo for washing the hair. Infusion of the dried tops and roots diuretic, carminative, and stimulant.

Saponin in stem = 1; tannin in stem = 1; calcium oxalate in leaves and stem = 1 — 2; sulfur, leaves and stem = 1; fats in leaves = 1, stem = 2; formic acid in leaves and stem = 1.

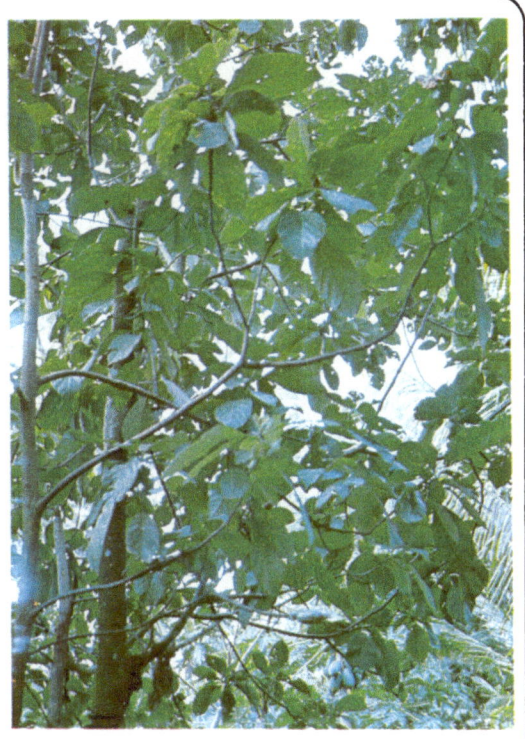

LAURACEAE
Persea americana Mill.
Abukado (Tag.); avocado, alligator pear (Engl.).

A tree, 10 m high or less. Leaves oblong to oval or obovate, about 20 cm long. Flowers in naked, panicled, pubescent cymes. Flowers small, the perianth-segments 4 to 5 mm long. Fruit large, fleshy, elongated, often some-what pear-shaped, 8 to 18 cm long, the flesh soft, edible, the single seed large.

A native of tropical America, it is a highly prized fruit in the Philippines.

Tea from avocado leaves is excellent for headache, fatigue, diseases of the throat and stomach, bronchial swellings, neuralgia and irregular menstrua-tion. Warm avocado leaves may be placed directly on the forehead to relieve neuralgia and headaches. Avocado seeds, roasted and ground, are used against the retention of urine and dysentery; the powder may be used as poultice over inflammations; an ointment of the pulverized seeds is sometimes em-ployed as a rubefacient, and a decoction of them, or a piece of a seed placed in the cavity of a tooth, is believed to cure toothache.

Saponin in leaves = 1, stem = 1 − 2; tannin, leaves = 1 − 2, stem = 2 − 3; glycosides in leaves and stem = 1; fats in stem = 1 − 2; formic acid in leaves and stem = 2.

19

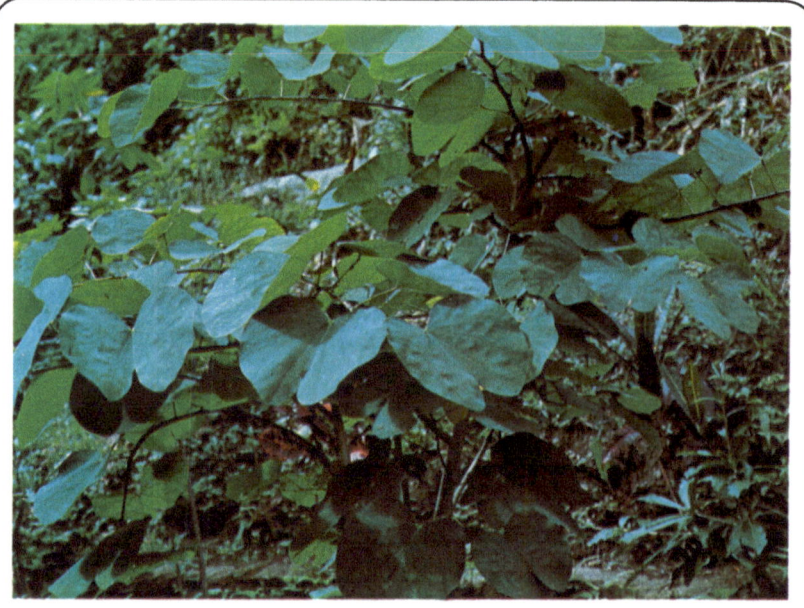

LEGUMINOSAE
Piliostigma malabaricum (Roxb.) Benth.
var. *acidum* (Korth.) de Wit
Alibangbang (Tag., Bis., Pamp.); *alambangbang* (Tag.); *balibamban* (Pamp.);
Kalibanbang (Pang., Tag.); *kalibanbang* (Ilk.); malabar Orchid (Engl.).

Small-sized but stocky tree reaching a height of 8 to 10 meters, with yellowish-brown, checked bark. Branches are freely rebranched forming a dense crown, the ultimate ones being smooth. Leaves, broader than long, 5 to 10 cm in length, heart-shaped at the base, and deeply notched at the apex. Flowers white and rather large. Pods are long, narrow, and flattened, 20 to 30 cm by 1.8 to 2.5 cm.

Very common in open, dry slopes in regions subject to a long· dry season in Luzon. It also occurs in India to Indo-China, Java; and Timor.

Infusion of the fresh flowers is antidysenteric. A decoction of the root-bark is a common remedy for liver trouble. Bark decoction is also considered antidysenteric; leaves are used in topicals applied on the head in fevers which are accompanied by headache.

Saponin in leaves and stem $= 1$; tannin in leaves and stem $= 1 - 2$; glycosides in stem $= 1$; calcium oxalate in leaves and stem $= 2 - 3$; fats in leaves $= 1$; peroxidase in leaves and stem $= 1 - 2$; phytosterol in leaves and stem $= 1$.

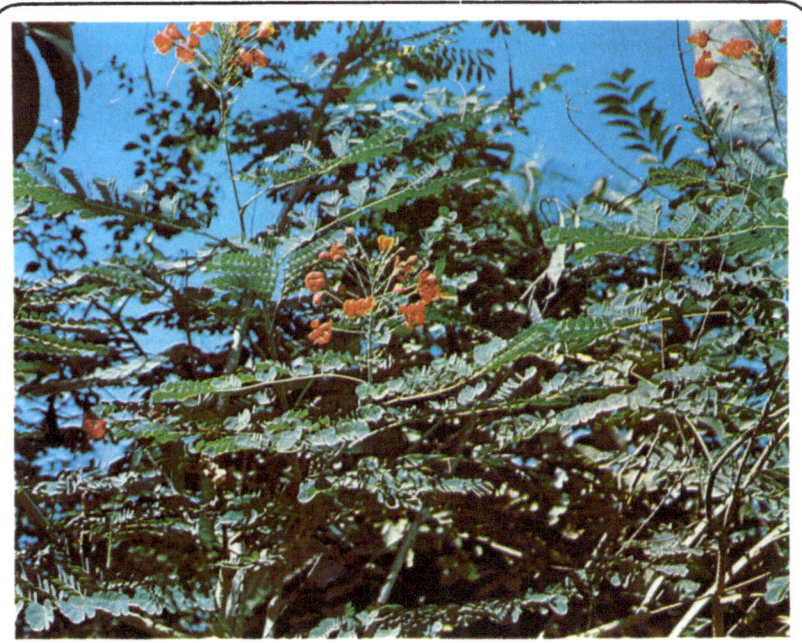

LEGUMINOSAE
Caesalpinia pulcherrima (L.) Sw.
Bulaklak ng paraiso (Tag.); *caballero* (Sp.); paradise flower, peacock flower (Engl.).

An erect, glabrous sparingly spiny shrub or small tree, 1.5 to 8 m high. Leaves bipinnate, pinnae 4 to 8 pairs, 6 to 12 cm long; leaflets sessile, 7 to 11 pairs, obtuse, elliptic, 1 to 2 cm long. Racemes terminal lax, the pedicels long, slender. Flowers red and yellow, or yellow, about 4 cm in diameter, the petals crisped, clawed; stamens long-exserted. Pods 5 to 9 cm long, 1.5 cm wide.

Commonly cultivated for ornamental purposes; native of tropical America.

Plant decoction or infusion purgative and emmenagogue. Decoction of the leaves for liver affections and as a wash for ulcers of the mouth and throat. Infusion of the leaves, roots or bark are employed for colds and skin diseases and are even said to induce abortion. Root decoction is used for the cure of intermittent fever. A decoction of the flowers is a popular remedy for erysipelas and for inflammation of the eyes, also used as tonic. Seeds are used as an effective abortifacient. Fruit astringent and is employed against diarrhea and dysentery.

Alkaloids in leaves and stem = 1 − 2; saponin in leaves = 1, stem = 2; tannin in leaves = 1 − 2, stem = 2 − 3; glucosides in leaves and stem = 1; calcium oxalate, leaves and stem = 2.

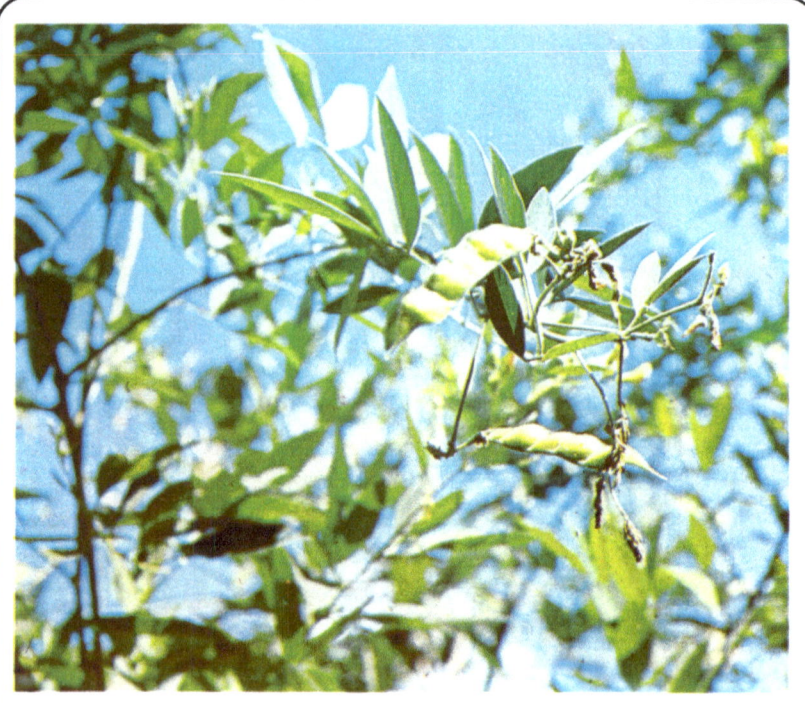

LEGUMINOSAE
Cajanus cajan (L.) Huth
Kagios, kalios, kadios, gablas (Tag.); *kaldis, kidis* (Ilk.); *tabios* (Bik., Bis.);
pigeon pea (Engl.).

An erect, branched, pubescent, shrubby plant, 1 to 2 m high. Leaflets 3,
oblong-lanceolate to oblanceolate, acuminate, 3 to 10 cm long, grayish
beneath when dry. Inflorescence axillary, of few-flowered, corymbose, peduncled racemes 3 to 7 cm long. Flowers yellow, about 1.5 cm long. Pods 4
to 7 cm long, about 1 cm wide, pubescent, prominently acuminate, obliquely
sulcate between the 2 to 7 seeds.

    Cultivated for its edible seeds; widely distributed in the Philippines;
cultivated and subspontaneous.

    Decoction or infusion of the leaves is used for coughs, diarrhea, and
abdominal trouble. Young leaves are chewed for sores in the mouth. Pulped
leaves are applied to sores. Expressed juice is given with a little salt in jaundice. Roots are thought to possess anthelmintic, sedative, expectorant and
vulnerary properties. Poultice of the seeds reduce swellings.

    Tannin in leaves and stem = 1; calcium oxalate, leaves and stem = 1;
sulfur, leaves and stem = 1; peroxidase in stem = 1; pectic substances in
stem = 1; protein, leaves and stem = 1 − 2.

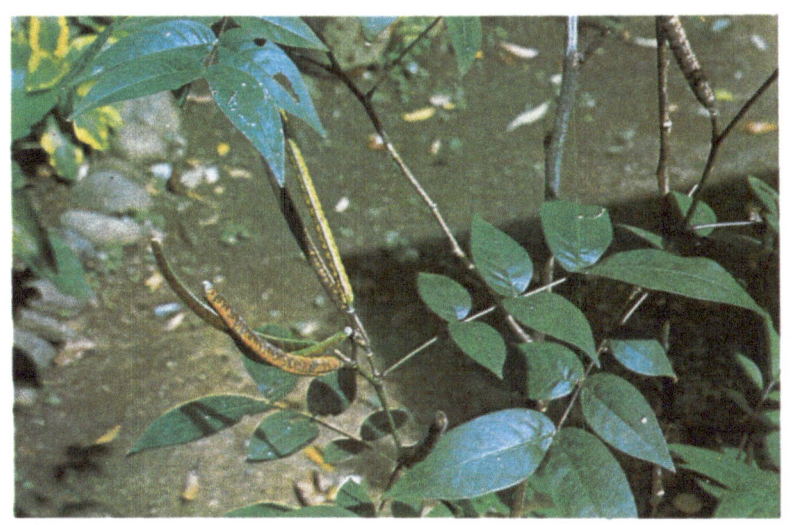

LEGUMINOSAE
Cassia occidentalis L.
Balatong-aso, kabal-kabalan, tambalisa (Tag.); *andadasi* (Ilk.); *Duda, sumting* (Bis.); coffee senna (Engl.).

An erect, somewhat branched, glabrous, suffrutescent herb or a shrubby plant, 0.8 to 1.5 m high. Leaves pinnate, about 20 cm long, the rachis with a large gland at the base. Leaflets rank-smelling, 5-pairs, oblong-lanceolate, acuminate, 4 to 9 cm long. Racemes few-flowered, axillary and terminal, corymbose. Flowers yellow, 2 cm long. Pods about 10 cm long, 9 mm wide, thickened, containing about 40 seeds.

Widely distributed in the Philippines, in open waste places. A native of tropical America.

The plant is reputed to possess tonic, diuretic, stomachic, and febrifuge properties. It is employed especially for dropsy, rheumatism, and venereal diseases. The plant in the form of an ointment is a remedy for ringworm, eczema, and other skin diseases. For snakebites, pounded fresh plant is applied as poultice. Leaves are used as a poultice to combat irritation and eczema. Leaf infusion purgative and antiherpetic. Roots are used as an anthelmintic. The seeds are the most active part of the plant and readily act as an emeto-cathartic; are also employed as a febrifuge, usually as an infusion with coffee. The seeds possess antiperiodic properties analogous to quinine. Entire plant or seed decoction remedy for constipation, indigestion, gastric pains and asthma. Seeds are sometimes employed as substitute for coffee.

Saponin in stem = 1; tannin in stem = 1; glycosides in stem = 1; sulfur in leaves and stem = 1; calcium oxalate in leaves and stem = 1 − 2; peroxidase in leaves and stem = 1

23

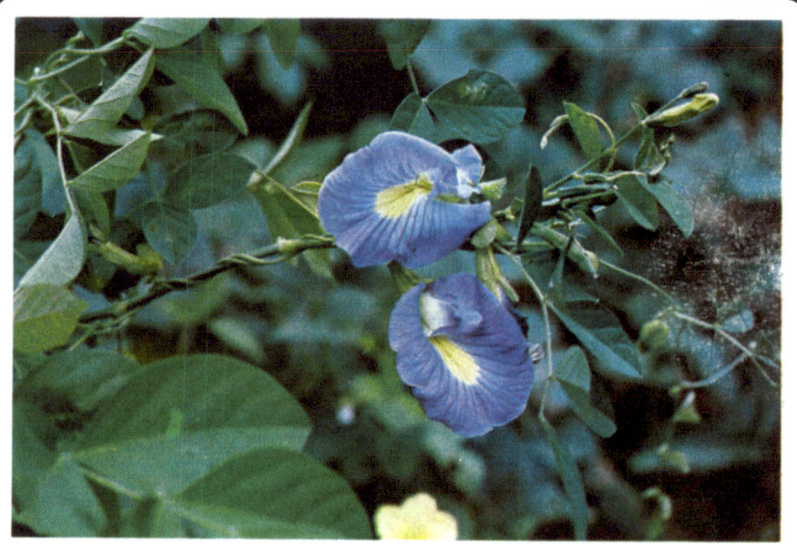

LEGUMINOSAE
Clitoria ternatea L.
Pukinggan, kolokanting (Tag.); *samsampin (Pang.); kalompagi* (Ilk.); *giting-princesa* (Bik.); *balog-balog* (Bis.); blue pea (Engl.).

A scandent vine, the stems sometimes 1 cm in diameter. Leaflets 5 to 7, elliptic to oblong, obtuse, 3 to 7 cm long, the stipels small, acicular. Flowers solitary, the bracts oblong, about 2 mm long, the bracteoles green, roundish, 5 to 8 mm long. Calyx green, 1.5 cm long. Corolla 3.5 to 4 cm long, the standard deep blue with a white or yellowish center, pale-blue or nearly white. Pod 5 to 10 cm long, flat, 6 to 10 seeded.

Quite common in thickets, often cultivated; throughout the Philippines.

The roots, taken as a purgative, were reported as toxic. The salient features of this poisoning, which is narcotic, consists of a) unconsciousness attended with extreme irritability and b) peculiar loss of memory. It is also considered aperient and diuretic. Root decoction is used to remove phlegm in chronic bronchitis and to bring nausea and vomiting when necessary. Root-bark infusion is used as a demulcent for irritation of the bladder and urethra; an alcoholic extract has been used as a cathartic. The leaves are used as poultice for swollen joints. Juice of the leaves mixed with common salt is applied warm all around the ear in carache, especially when accompanied with swelling of the neighboring glands. Seeds are considered anthelmintic and are used as a mild purgative.

Alkaloids in leaves and stem = 1 − 2; calcium oxalate, leaves and stem = 1; sulfur in stem = 1, fats in leaves and stem = 1; pectic substances in stem = 1.

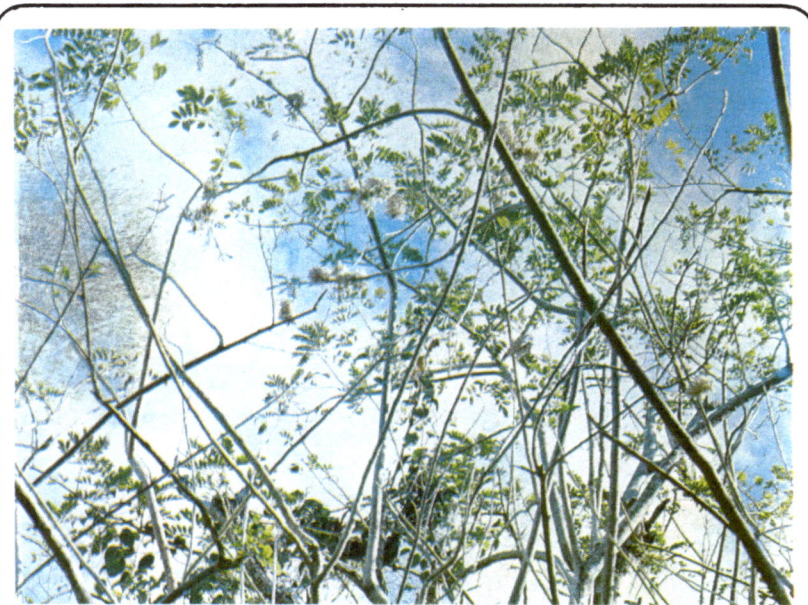

LEGUMINOSAE
Gliricidia sepium (Jacq.) Steud.
Madre cacao, cacauate (Sp. Tag.); *marikakau, kakauati* (Tag.).

A glabrous deciduous tree, 3 to 10 m high. Leaves 15 to 25 cm long; leaflets about 13, opposite, oblong-ovate, slightly acuminate, blunt, base usually rounded, 4 to 6 cm long, rather pale beneath, green and shining on the upper surface. Racemes numerous on the leaflets branches; densely many-flowered, solitary in the axils of fallen leaves, 4 to 8 cm long. Flowers 2 cm long, pink, the calyx truncate. Standard reflexed, retuse, pale-yellow in the median part. Pods narrowly oblong to lanceolate, 10 to 14 cm long, about 2 cm wide, flat, 6 to 8-seeded, dehiscent.

In thickets, hedge rows, etc., throughout the Philippines in and about towns; a native of Mexico.

Juice of the leaves, bark, and roots is used to cure itches and wounds and the crushed leaves are applied to rheumatic pains and to fractures.

The wood of kakauati is hard and durable, being used locally for small house posts, agricultural implement, tool handles, etc. The leaves have a fetid smell and are often used externally to rid dogs of ticks and fleas, and cattle of ticks.

Saponin in stem = 1; tannin in leaves and stem = 1; glucosides in leaves and stem = 1; calcium oxalate in stem = 1; sulfur, leaves and stem = $1 - 2$; peroxidase in stem = $1 - 2$; fats, leaves.

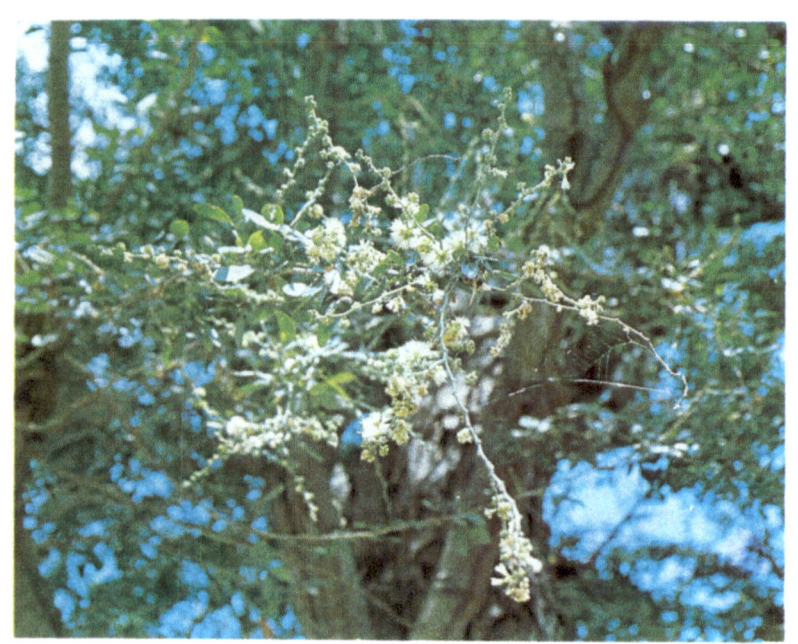

LEGUMINOSAE
Pithecellobium dulce (Roxb.) Benth.
Kamachili (Tag., Bik.); *kamansile, kamachilis* (Tag.); *damortis* (Ilk.); *kamantilis* (Pang.); *komonsili, kamunsil* (Bis.).

A tree, 5 to 18 m high, the ultimate branches often pendulous, armed with short, sharp, stipular spines. Leaves evenly 2-pinnate, 4 to 8 cm long; pinnae a single pair, each pinna bearing a single pair of oblique, ovate-oblong, obtuse, 1 to 4 cm long leaflets. Flowers white, in dense heads about 1 cm in diameter, their peduncles solitary or fascicled in the axils of small bracts, along the slender branchlets. Pod turgid, twisted, often spiral, 10 to 18 cm long, about 1 cm wide, dehiscent along the lower suture, the valves red when ripe. Seeds 6 to 8, surrounded by an edible, whitish, pulpy arillus.

Common and widely distributed. A native of tropical America.

The leaves, when applied as plasters, allay pain, even those of venereal sores, and relieve convulsions. The leaves, with salt, cure indigestion and also produce abortion; the root-bark is good for dysentery. Bark is also used for tanning.

Tannin in leaves and stem = $1 - 2$; calcium oxalate, leaves and stem = 1; peroxidase in stem = 1; pectic substances, leaves and stem = 1; hydrocellulose in leaves and stem = 1

26

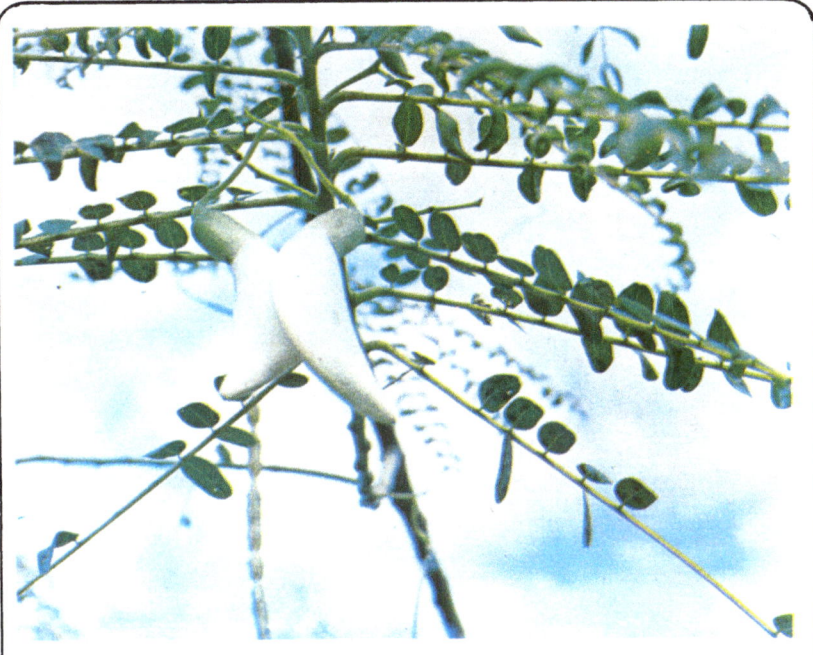

LEGUMINOSAE
Sesbania grandiflora (Linn.) Pers.
Katurai (Tag., Pang.); *katodai* (Ilk.); *gauai-gauai* (Bis.).

The tree is 5 to 12 m in height. The leaves 20 to 30 cm long, pinnate, having 20 to 40 pairs of leaflets, which are 2.5 to 3.5 cm long. Racemes short, axillary. Flowers few, very large, white, 7 to 9 cm long. Calyx green, subtruncate or very shallowy 2-lipped. Pods pendulous, linear, 20 to 60 cm long, 7 to 8 mm wide, somewhat curved, many seeded.

Common cultivated; throughout the Philippines.

The root of the red-flowered variety, rubbed into a paste with water, is applied for rheumatism. The juice of the root is given with honey as an expectorant in catarrh. The bark is very astringent and an infusion of it is given in smallpox and other eruptive fevers; also considered tonic and febrifuge; given in diarrhea and dysentery. The juice of the leaves and flowers is used as a popular remedy for nasal catarrh and headache. The leaves are said to be aperient, diuretic. The edible flowers are considered emollient and laxative.

Saponin in leaves and stems = $1 - 2$; tannin, leaves and stem = $1 - 2$; glycosides in leaves = 1; calcium oxalate in stem = 1; sulfur in stem = $1 - 2$; peroxidase in leaves = 1, stem = 2.

27

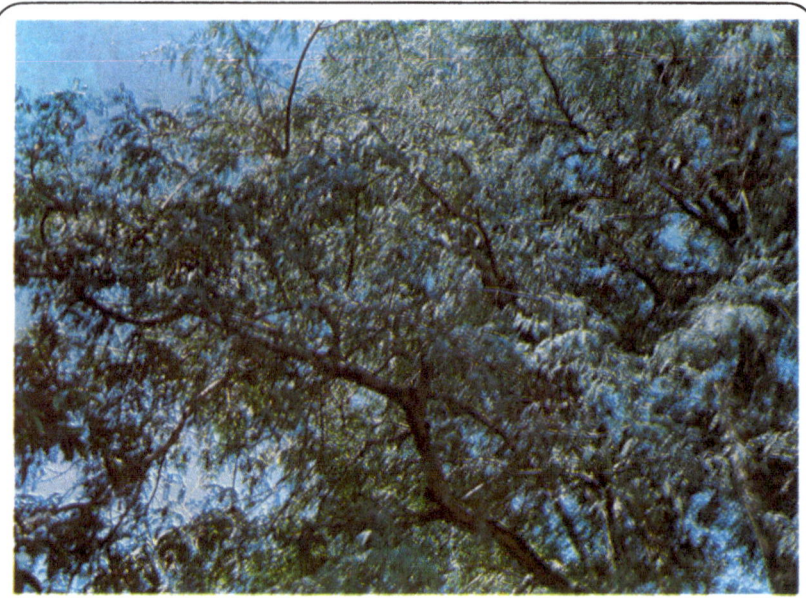

LEGUMINOSAE
Tamarindus indica L.*
Sampalok (Tag.); *tamarindo* (Sp.); *sambag* (Bis.); *salomague* (Ilk.); *sambak, sambalagi* (Bik.); tamarind (Engl.).

A large tree, 12 to 20 m high, nearly glabrous. Leaves even-pinnate, 6 to 10 cm long; leaflets 20 to 40, rather close, oblong, obtuse, 1 to 2 cm long. Racemes mostly axillary, sometimes panicled, 5 to 10 cm long. Calyx about 1 cm long. Petals yellowish with pink stripes, obovate-oblong, less than 1 cm long. Pods oblong, thickened, 6 to 15 cm long, 2 to 3 cm wide, slightly compressed, crustaceous, the mesocarp pulpy, acid, edible.

Widely distributed in the Philippines.

Young leaves are used in fomentations for rheumatism, and are applied to sores and wounds, as a poultice for inflammations of the ankles, joints, etc. to reduce swelling and to relieve pain, as a sweetened leaf decoction is good for cough, a filtered hot juice of young leaves is used for conjunctivitis. As a decoction is anthelmintic, useful for jaundice, and pounded as application to erysipelas. The bark is astringent and tonic, the ash of the bark is given internally as digestive, in lotions and in poultice relieves sores, ulcers, boils, and caterpillar rash, as a decoction for asthma, amenorrhea and as febrifuge. The pulp is used as a mild laxative; also for scurvy. A poultice of the flowers is said to be helpful in inflammatory affections of the conjunctiva. Powdered seeds are given in dysentery and diarrhea.

Saponin in stem = 1; tannin in leaves and stem = 1 − 2; glucosides in leaves and stem = 1; peroxidase, leaves and stem = 1 − 2; fats in stem = 1.

28

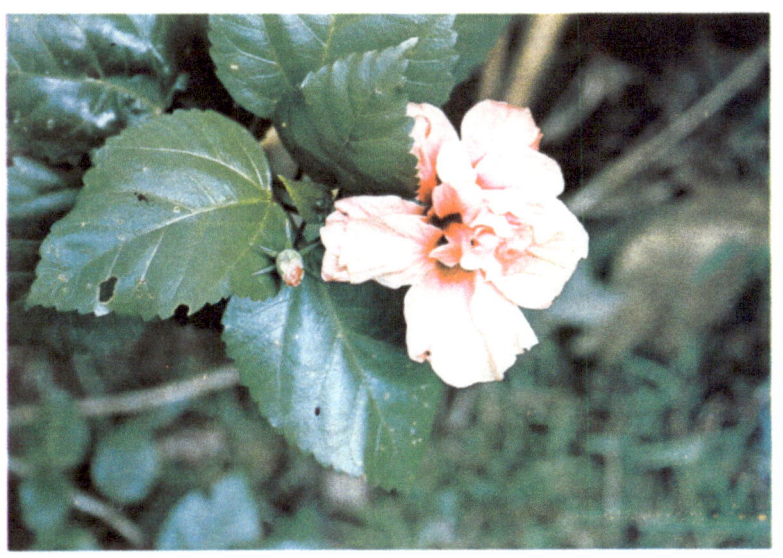

MALVACEAE
Hibiscus rosa-sinensis L.
Gumamela (Tag.); *gumamela* (Tag., Bis., Pamp.); *kayanga* (Ilk.; Bik., Bis.);
aratongan (Pamp.); Hibiscus, china rose, shoeflower (Engl.).

An erect, much-branched, glabrous shrub, 1 to 4 m high. Leaves ovate,
acuminate, coarsely toothed, 7 to 12 cm long. Flowers solitary, axillary, very
large, about 10 cm long, 12 cm in diameter. Bracteoles 6, lanceolate, green, 8
mm long or less. Calyx green, 2 cm long, the lobes ovate. Petals red, obovate,
rounded, imbricate. Staminal-tube slender, longer than the corolla.

    Commonly cultivated; probably a native of South-eastern Asia.

    The plant possesses anti-infection and anti-inflammation properties.
Decoction of dried plant is used for infection of urinary tract. Roots, barks,
leaves, and flowers in decoction are used as emollient. Fresh leaves are
crushed and applied as poultice to abscesses and carbuncles. The bark is used
as an emmenagogue. Flower buds, beaten into a paste, are applied as poultice
to boils, cancerous swellings and mumps. The red flowers regulate menstruation; they are somewhat purgative and are sometimes said to cause abortion.
Infusion of flowers used as an expectorant in bronchitis. Decoction of flowers
effective for coughs. The dark red petals are administered in the form of a
mucilaginous infusion in irritable conditions of the genito-urinary tract; also a
refrigerant drink in fevers. The seeds, pounded into a pulp and mixed with
water, are given with much benefit in gonorrhea. Decoction of roots is used
for sore eyes.

    Calcium oxalate, leaves and stem = 1 − 2; sulfur in stem = 1; peroxidase
in leaves and stem = 1 − 2; fats, leaves and stem = 1 − 2; protein, leaves
and stem = 1 − 2.

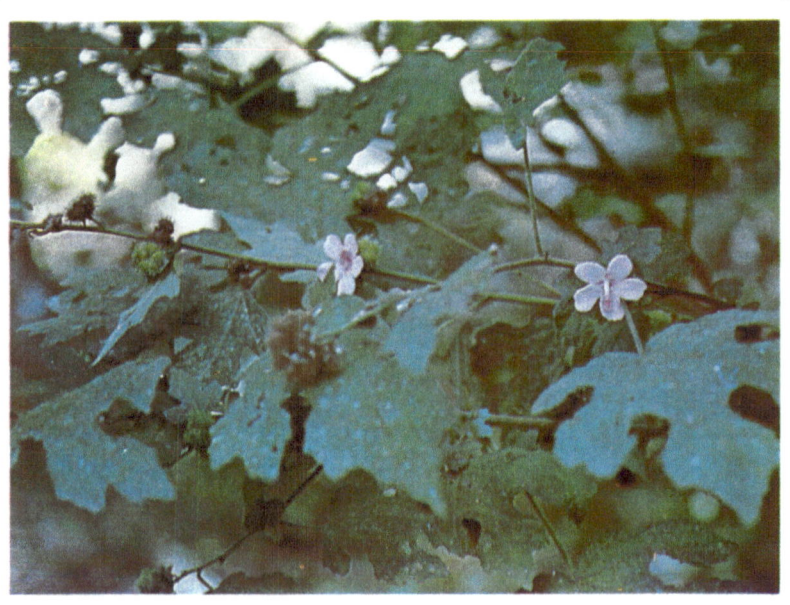

MALVACEAE
Urena lobata L.
Kulutkulutan, mangkit, palisin (Tag.); *dalupang* (Tag., Bis., Pamp.); *baranggot* (Bik.); *kulit* (Pang.); *kulukulut* (Ilk.).

An erect, branched, shrubby plant, 0.6 to 2.5 m high, exceedingly variable, more or less pubescent. Leaves pale beneath, ovate to sub-orbicular, 3 to 9 cm long, cordate, more or less toothed or somewhat lobed or angled, the lobes not extending beyond the middle of the leaf, the sinuses usually broad, acute. Flowers axillary, solitary or somewhat fascicled, pink, about 1.7 mm in diameter. Fruit depressed-globose, about 7 mm in diameter, the 5 carpels covered with short, retrorsely barbed spines.

Widely distributed in the Philippines.

The root as a decoction relieves colic; is used in dysentery, acute tonsilitis and tetanus, infusion is emollient and refrigerant, for skin diseases which are accompanied by smarting and inflammation. Fresh leaves are applied as poultice in sprains and bruises and in poisonous snake bites; boiled and pounded as a poultice in inflammations of the intestines and bladder. Flowers are employed as an expectorant. A decoction of the seeds taken internally is an effective vermifuge.

The bast fiber of this plant is of the jute type and is said to be more easily extracted than jute. The rope made from the fibers is fairly strong. In other countries, the product is used as cordage material.

Tannin in leaves and stem = 1 − 2; glycosides, leaves and stem = 1; calcium oxalate in leaves and stem = 1 − 2; sulfur in leaves and stem = 1 − 2; peroxidase, leaves and stem = 1 − 2.

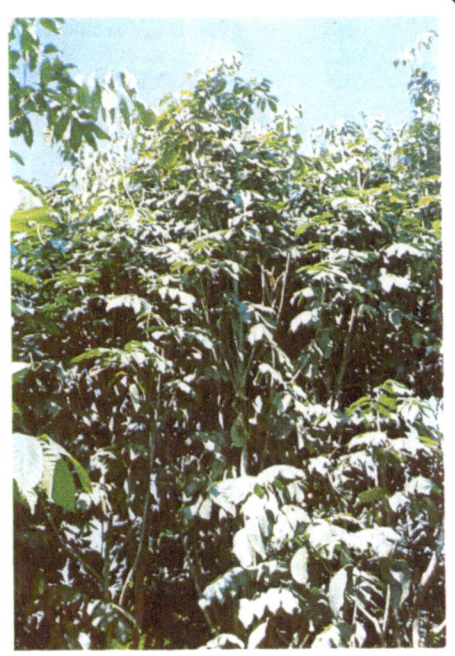

MELIACEAE
Lansium domesticum Corr.
Lansones (Tag.); *tubua* (Bik.); *bukan, bulahan, boboa* (Bis.).

A tree, 4 to 8 m high or more, slightly pubescent or nearly glabrous. Leaves alternate, 20 to 40 cm long; leaflets 5 - 7, oblong or elliptic-oblong, acuminate, 7 to 18 cm long, the nerves prominent on the lower surface. Perfect flowers sessile, small, in spikes which are solitary or fascicled on the trunk and larger branches, much shorter than the leaves. Fruit edible, oblong-ovate or ellipsoid, pubescent, usually about 3 cm long, the pericarp tough. Seeds 1 or 2, surrounded by translucent pulp, as are the remaining 3 or 4 aborted seeds.

Widely distributed in the Philippines in cultivation.

The bark is astringent and its decoction is used for dysentery; powdered, it is a remedy for scorpion stings. The seeds, ground and mixed with water, are given to children as vermifuge; also as an antipyretic. The resin from the bark is prescribed for flatulence, for swellings and as an antispasmodic. A tincture prepared from the dried rind, is useful as an antidiarrhetic. The dried fruit peel, when burned, makes a pleasant inhalant in a sick room, and gives an aromatic smell which drives away mosquitoes.

Saponin in leaves and stem = 1 − 2; tannin in leaves = 1; stem = 2 − 3; calcium oxalate in leaves = 1, stem = 2 − 3; fats in leaves and stem = 1; sulfur in leaves and stem = 1; peroxidase in leaf and stem = 1.

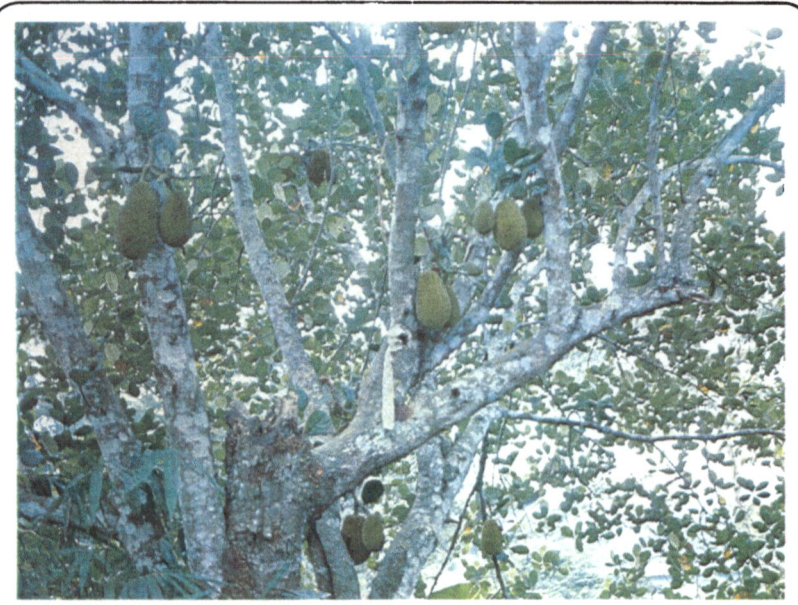

MORACEAE
Artocarpus heterophyllus Lmk.
Langka or *nangka* (Tag., Ilk., Bis); jack fruit (Engl.).

A smooth tree, attaining a height of from 8 to 15 meters. The leaves are alternate, leathery, elliptic-oblong to obovate, entire or sometimes 3-lobed, 7 to 15 cm long; the apex and base are both pointed. The female heads embraced by spathaceous, deciduous, stipular sheaths, 5 to 8 cm long. The sepals two, spikes 5 to 15 cm long. The fruit greenish-yellow or very green when ripe, fleshy, hanging on short stalks from the main stem or from large branches in old trees, oblong, 25 to 60 cm long, and covered with pyramidal projections. The seeds numerous, oblong, 2.5 to 4 cm long. The testa thin, coriaceous, and surrounded by luscious pulp which is edible.

Cultivated throughout the Philippines at low and medium altitude, and in some regions is spontaneous.

Ash of the leaves is applied on wounds and ulcers as cicatrizant. Root decoction for diarrhea and fever. The milky juice of the tree is used in glandular swellings and snake bites; mixed with vinegar and applied to these swellings and to abscesses, it promotes suppuration. Ripe fruit demulcent, nutritive and laxative. The starch of the seed is given in bilious colic. Roasted seeds have an aphrodisiac action.

Alkaloids in leaves = 1 − 2, stem = 1; saponin in leaves and stem = 1 − 2; glucosides in leaves and stem = 1; tannin in leaves and stem = 1; calcium oxalate in leaves = 1, stem = 2 − 3.

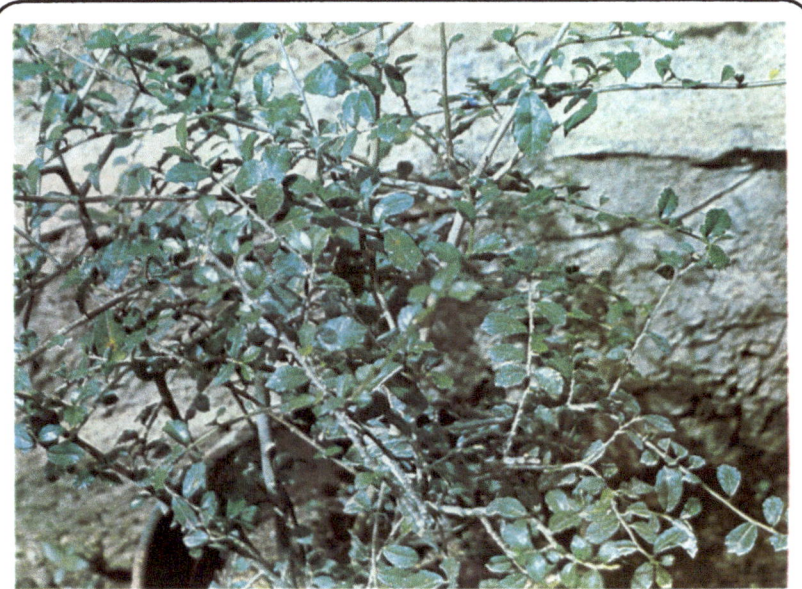

MORACEAE
Streblus asper Lour.
Calios (Tag.); *aludig* (Ilk.); *ampas* (Pamp.); *bagtak* (Bis.).

A rigid, densely branched tree, 4 to 15 m high. Leaves oblong-ovate to sub-rhomboid, very scabrid, 4 to 12 cm long, finely toothed, obtuse to acuminate, base narrowed. Male heads solitary or in pairs, 4 to 7 mm in diameter, short-peduncled, globose, greenish-yellow or nearly white. Female flowers peduncled, usually in pairs, green, the sepals accrescent and nearly enclosing the fruit. Fruit ovoid, pale yellow, 8 to 10 mm long, the pericarp soft, fleshy, the seed 5 to 6 mm long, ovoid.

Very common in the Philippines.

Bark decoction is used for disinfecting wounds, internally used for skin diseases called "culebra", for fever, dysentery, and diarrhea. Bark is chewed as an antidote in snake poisoning. Root is used in epilepsy and inflammatory swellings and is applied to boils; juice is astringent and antiseptic. The latex is applied to sore heels and chapped hands, on glandular swellings.

Glucosides in stem = 1; calcium oxalate in leaves and stem = 1 − 2; sulfur. leaves and stem = 2; peroxidase in leaves and stem = 1; hydrocellulose, leaves and stem = 1 − 2.

33

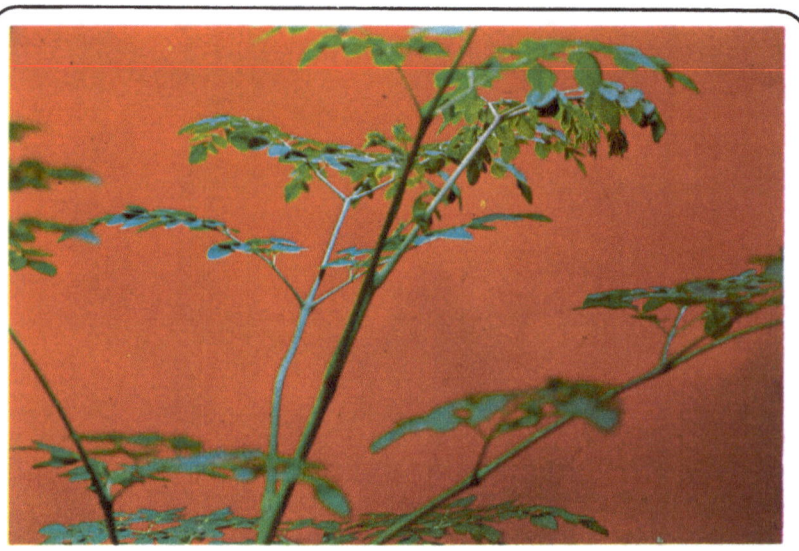

MORINGACEAE
Moringa oleifera Lam.
Malunggay (Tag.); *arunggai* (Pang.); *balungai* (Bis.); *dool* (Bis., Pamp.); *Marunggay* (Ilk.); horse-radish tree (Engl.).

A small tree, 8 m high or less, bark corky, roots with a pungent taste. Leaves 25 to 50 cm long, usually 3-pinnate; pinnae 4-6 pairs; leaflets 3-9 on the ultimate pinnules, pale beneath, thin, ovate to elliptic, 1 to 2 cm long. Panicles spreading. Flowers white, 1.5 to 2 cm long. Fertile filaments villous at the base. Ovary hairy. Pod 15 to 30 cm long, pendulous, 3-angled, 9-ribbed. Seeds 3-angled, winged on the angles.

Widely distributed in the Philippines; a native of India.

Leaves are used as galactagogue; as a poultice in reducing glandular swellings; it is also said to have purgative properties. The root, if chewed and applied to the bite of a snake, will prevent the poison from spreading; is regarded as an acrid, pungent remedy which is stimulant and diuretic; as a decoction for hiccoughs, asthma, gout, lumbago, rheumatism, enlarged spleen or liver and internal and deep-seated inflammations, as an effective gargle, and as fomentation to relieve spasms. The pods have anthelmintic properties and are administered in affections of the liver and spleen, in articular pains etc.

Tannin in stem = 2, sulfur in stem = $1 - 2$; calcium oxalate in leaves and stem = $1 - 2$; peroxidase in stem = 2; pectic substances, leaves and stem = 1.

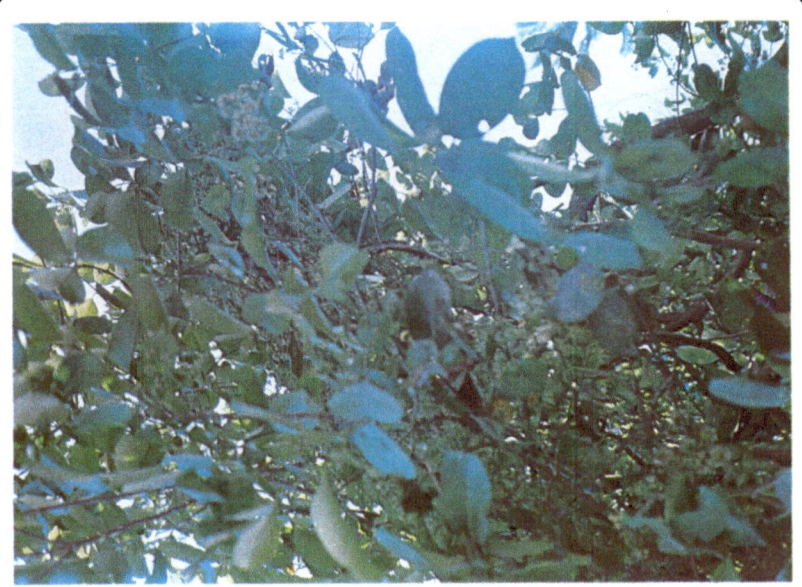

MYRTACEAE

Syzygium cuminii (Linn.) Skeels

Duhat (Tag., Bis.); *duat-nasi* (Pamp.); *lomboi* (Ilk., Pamp., Tag., Bis.); *longboi* (Ilk.); black plum, Java plum (Engl.).

A smooth tree, 4 to 15 m in height. Leaves leathery oblong-ovate to elliptic or obovate and 6 to 12 cm long, the tip being broad and shortly pointed. The panicles are borne mostly from the branchlets below the leaves, often being axillary or terminal, and are 4 to 6 cm long. The flowers numerous, scented, pink or nearly white, without stalks, and borne in crowded fascicles on the ends of the branchlets. The calyx is funnel-shaped, about 4 mm long, and 4-toothed. The petals cohere and fall all together as a small disk. The stamens are very numerous and about as long as the calyx. Fruit oval to elliptic, 1.5 to 3.5 cm long, dark purple or nearly black, luscious, fleshy and edible; it contains a single large seed.

Throughout the Philippines; planted and spontaneous.

Leaves are used for poulticing skin complaints; root-bark decoction is administered in diarrhea. Bark decoction is given internally in dysentery; used as an enema to cleanse ulcers, and as a gargle. The ripe fruit is astringent and is considered an efficient remedy for diabetes mellitus. Wine prepared from the juice of the ripe fruit, is an agreeable stomachic and carminative; also diuretic.

Tannin in leaves and stem = $2 - 3$; glycosides, leaves and stem = 1; calcium oxalate in leaves and stem = $1 - 2$; sulfur in leaves = 2, stem = 1; fats from stem = 2; peroxidase in leaves and stem = $1 - 2$.

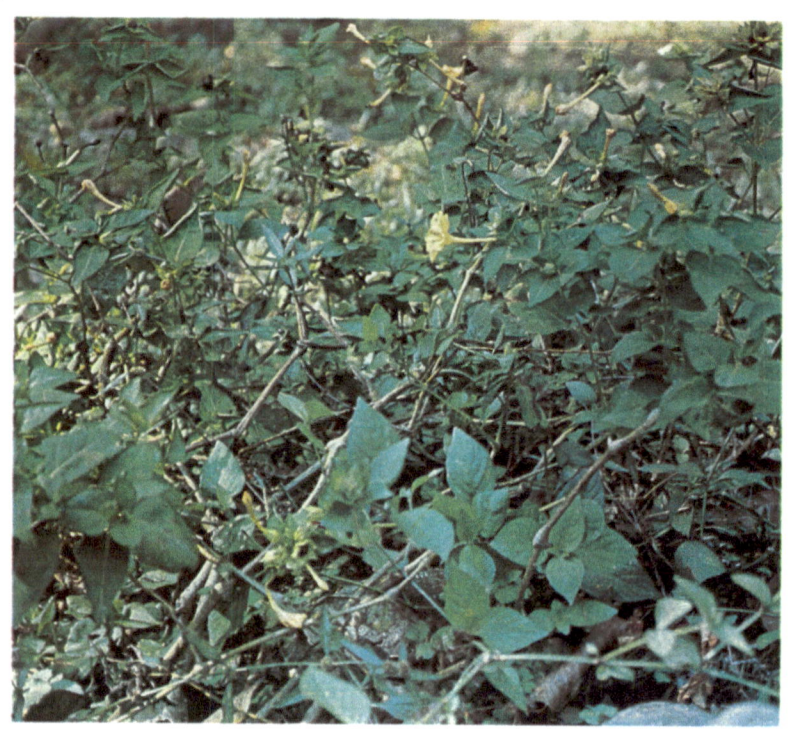

NYCTAGINACEAE
Mirabilis jalapa L.
Alas cuatro, oraciones (Tag., Sp.); *gilala* (Tag.); Four o'clock, Marvel of Peru (Engl.).

An erect, nearly or quite glabrous, branched plant, 20 to 80 cm high. Leaves 4 to 10 cm long, narrowly ovate, acuminate, base often subtruncate, and somewhat inequilateral. Involucres crowded, calyx-like 1 cm long or less, 1-flowered. Perianth white, purple, or yellow, the tube cylindric, slightly enlarged upward, 3 to 4 cm long, the limb spreading. Fruit narrowly ovoid, about 8 mm long, black, finely ribbed.

Cultivated throughout the Philippines; a native of tropical America.

The bruised leaves are used for poulticing boils and abscesses; leaf infusion is prescribed as a diuretic and for dropsy, the juice is used for uterine discharges. The roots have been reported as mild purgative and as emeto-cathartic.

Alkaloid in leaves and stem = 1; saponin in leaves and stem = 1 − 2; calcium oxalate, leaves, stem and root = 2; fats in leaves and stem = 1, root = 1 − 2; formic acid in leaves and stem = 1, root = 2; pectic substances in leaves and stem = 1 − 2.

36

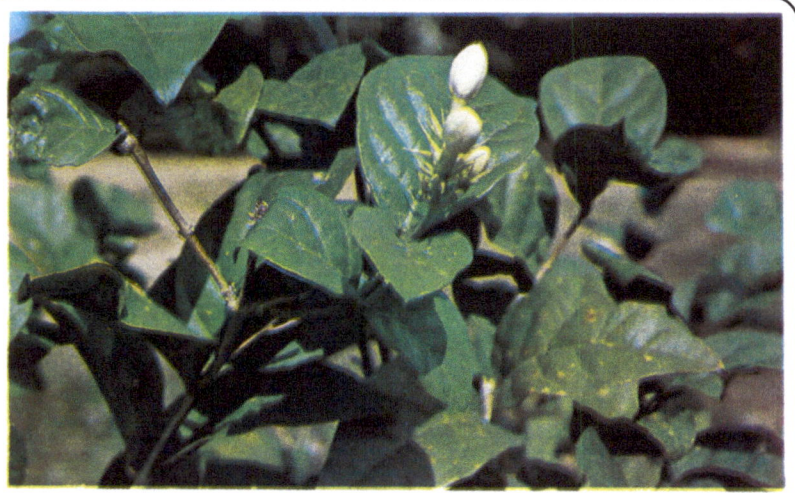

OLEACEAE
Jasminum sambac (Linn.) Ait.
Sampaguita (Tag., Sp.); *kampupot* (Pamp., Tag.); *manul* (Bis.); Arabian Jasmine, sambac (Engl.).

A spreading or sprawling, smooth shrub usually less than 2 m in height. Leaves glossy, ovate or rounded, and 6 to 12 cm long, with short stalks, pointed or blunt tip and pointed or rounded base. Flowers white, very fragrant, and borne singly or in threes on axillary or terminal inflorescences. The calyx-teeth are 8 to 10, very slender, and 5 to 8 mm long. The corolla tube is slender and 1 to 1.5 cm long; the limb is usually double and 1.5 to 2 cm in diameter. The double kind is called "kampupot" and this is less fragrant.

Commonly cultivated throughout the Philippines for ornamental purposes.

Dried leaves, soaked in water and made into a poultice, are applied to indolent ulcers; given internally in decoction for fever, are used for poulticing skin complaints and wounds. The leaves and flowers are considered lactiuge, being bruised and applied to the breasts. Flower decoction antispasmodic; also used as eyewash. The roots are said to be poisonous; tincture made from them is said to have very powerful sedative, anesthetic and vulnerary properties. For sprains and fractures, roots are used as external poultice. Decoction of roots or infusion of the flowers is employed in pulmonary catarrh, bronchitis, and also in asthma.

In China, the flowers are used for giving an aroma to tea. In Malaysia, women soak the flowers in water to be used for washing the face.

Tannin in stem = 1; glucosides in leaves and stem and root = 1; calcium oxalate in leaves = 3; iron in stem and root = 1; fats in flowers = 3; silicon in flowers = 2.

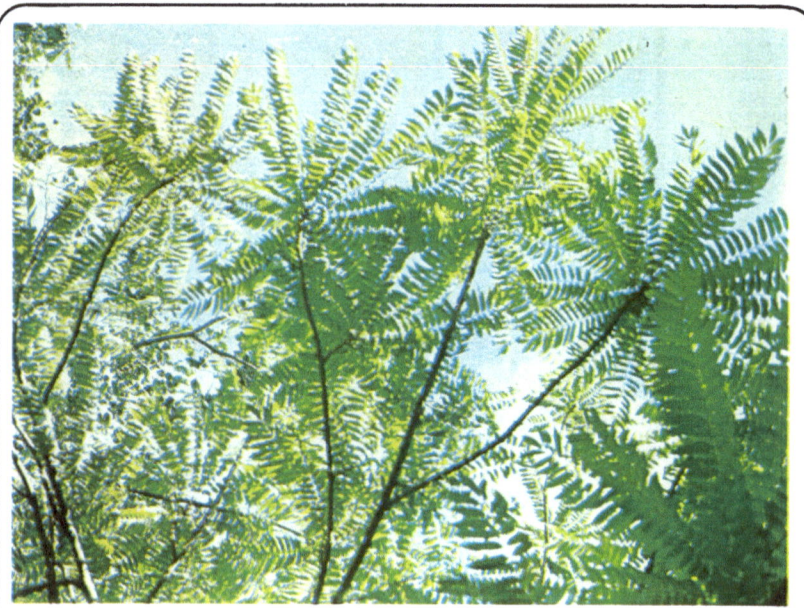

OXALIDACEAE
Averrhoa bilimbi L.
Kamias, iba, kalamias, kolonanas Tag.); *kilingiua* (Bis.); *pias* (Ilk.); *kiling-iba* (Bik.); bilimbi, cucumber tree (Engl.).

Small tree, 5 to 12 m high. Leaves pinnate, 20 to 60 cm long, the rachis and leaflets pubescent, leaflets 10 to 17 pairs, oblong, acuminate, 5 to 10 cm long. Panicles from the trunk and larger branches, usually fascicled, pubescent, 15 cm long or less. Flowers about 1.5 cm long, somewhat fragrant. Calyx pubescent. Corolla purple, often marked with white. Fruit subcylindric or with 5, obscure, broad, rounded, longitudinal lobes, green, acid, edible, about 4 cm long. Seeds not arillate.

Widely distributed in the Philippines; throughout the tropics; a native of tropical America.

Leaf decoction is given for inflammation of the rectum. As a paste, it is applied for mumps, rheumatism and pimples. Infusion of the flowers is used for coughs. The fruit is astringent stomachic and refrigerant. The juice of the fruit made into a syrup forms a cooling drink in fevers, antiscorbutic, and is also used in some slight cases of hemorrhage from the bowels, stomach, and internal hemorrhoids.

Saponin in stem = 1; tannin in leaves = 1, stem = 2; glucosides in stem = 1; calcium oxalate in stem = 1; sulfur in leaves = 1, stem = 2; peroxidase in stem = 2; formic acid in leaves and stem = 2.

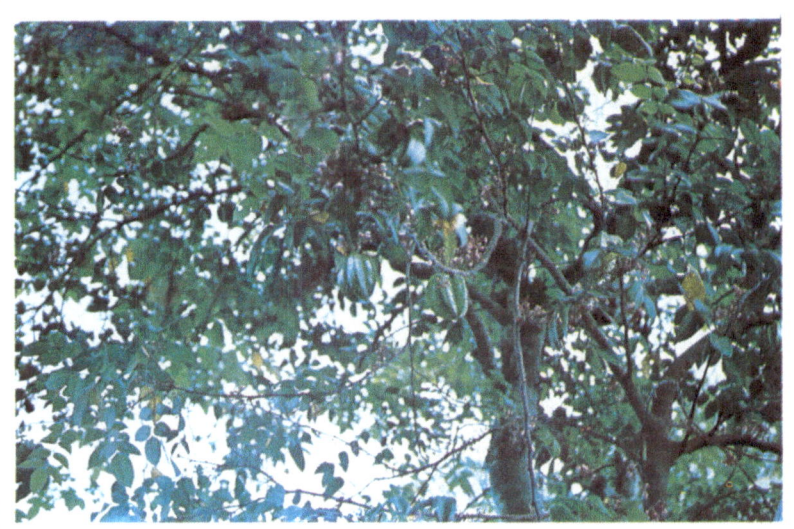

OXALIDACEAE
Averrhoa carambola L.
Balimbing (Tag., Bik.); *balingbing* (Bik., Bis.); *daligan* (Ilk.); *garahan* (Bis.); carambola (Engl.).

Shrub or small tree, 6 m high or less. Leaves pinnate, about 15 cm long, leaflets quite glabrous, usually about 5 pairs, ovate to ovate-lanceolate, acuminate, the upper ones about 5 cm long, the lower ones smaller. Panicles small, axillary, usually about 3 cm long. Flowers 5 to 6 mm long, somewhat campanulate. Calyx reddish-purple. Petals pale-purple to rather bright-purple, often margined with white. Stamens 10, the 5-shorter ones usually without anthers. Fruit fleshy, green or greenish-yellow usually about 6 cm long with 5 longitudinal, sharp, angular, lobes, acid, edible. Seeds arillate.

Widely distributed in the Philippines and throughout the tropics; a native of tropical America.

Crushed leaves or shoots are used as an application for chicken pox, ringworm and headache. The fruit is laxative, refrigerant, and antiscorbutic; stimulates appetite, is a febrifuge and antidysenteric. Infusion, decoction or tincture of the crushed seeds is emmenagogue, lactagogue, and abortifacient in large doses. The seed may be regarded as a narcotic and emetic. Powdered, it is a good anodyne in asthma, colic, jaundice and the infusion is similarly useful.

Alkaloids in leaves = 1 − 2; saponin in leaves and stem = 1 − 2; tannin in leaves and stem = 1 − 2; glucosides in leaves and stem = 1; calcium oxalate in leaves = 1, stem = 2; sulfur in leaves and stem = 2; formic acid, leaves and stem = 2 − 3; peroxidase in stem = 2.

39

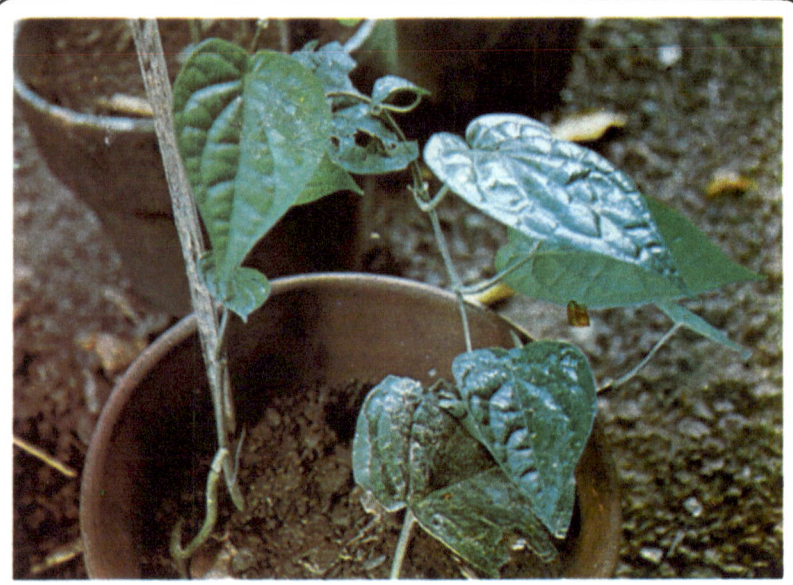

PIPERACEAE
Piper betle L.
Ikmo, itmo, buyo-anis (Tag.); *buyo, buyo-buyo* (Bik.); *gaued* (Ilk.); *kanisi, mamon* (Bis.); *samat* (Pamp.); betel, betel leaf pepper (Engl.).

A glabrous climbing vine reaching a height of 2 to 4 m. Upper leaves ovate, 10 to 13 cm long, mostly 7-nerved from near the base, the outer pair of nerves free to the base, apex acuminate, base somewhat inequilaterally rounded or cordate, the petioles 1.5 to 2.5 cm long, sheathing. Male spikes about as long as the leaves, about 2 mm in diameter, the rachis hirsute. Female spikes, when mature, red, fleshy, 2 to 4 cm long, 0.5 to 1 cm thick.

Common throughout the Philippines, wild and cultivated.

The fresh, crushed leaves are used as antiseptic for cuts and wounds, and as a poultice for boils, together with lime and betel nut, constitute a masticatory in general use among the Filipinos, who consider it a preservative of the teeth and a prophylactic against certain complaints of the stomach; with oil are used as a carminative medicine applied to the abdomen of children suffering from gastric disorders; a liquid extract is prescribed in catarrhal inflammations of the throat, larynx and bronchitis, and also in coughs, indigestion, and are also considered stimulant, astringent, aphrodisiac, stomachic and febrifuge. A warm poultice of the leaves and oil (coconut) is applied in the chest of children in catarrhal and pulmonary affections and is administered for congestion and other affections of the liver.

Alkaloid in leaves and stem = 2 − 3; tannin in stem = 1; peroxidase in stem = 1; fats, leaves and stem = 1; pectic substances in leaves = 1.

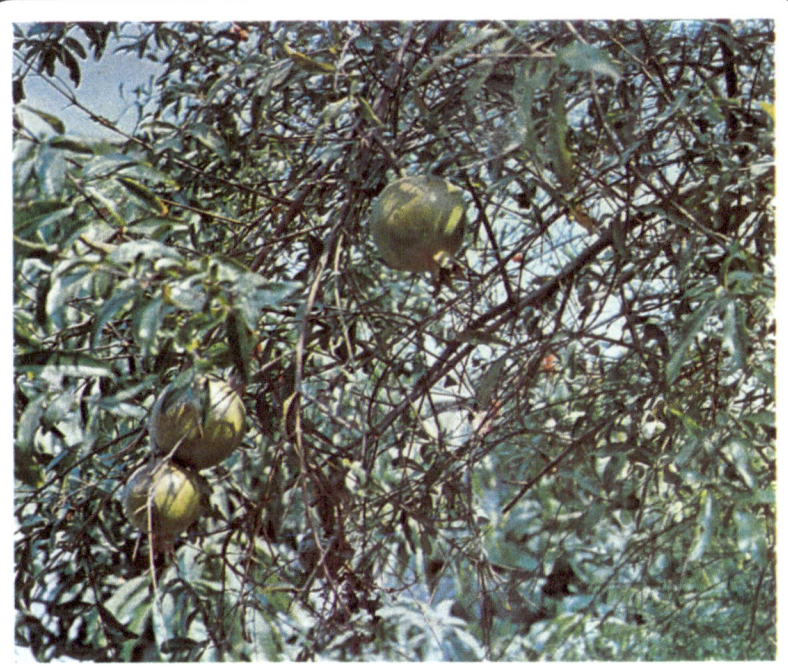

PUNICACEAE
Punica granatum L.
Granada (Tag., Sp.); pomegranate (Engl.).

A shrub, 2 to 3 m high, the branchlets slender, 4-angled, often terminating with a short spine. Leaves oblong-lanceolate to oblong elliptic, 4 to 6 cm long, short-petioled, acute or obtuse, narrowed at both ends. Flowers red, the calyx 2.5 to 3 cm long, the segments usually 6. Petals obovate, nearly 2 cm long. Fruit globose, reddish or purplish, about 5 cm in diameter, containing many seeds surrounded by a red pulp.

Occasionally cultivated in the Philippines.

Seeds are considered stomachic and the pulp is said to be cardiacal. The rind of the fruit is used internally in decoction as anthelmintic, in diarrhea, advanced stages of dysentery, and in other cases requiring the use of astringents. The root-bark, being the most astringent part of the plant, is a vermifuge. The bark and flowers are prescribed against hemorrhage; powdered flower buds are useful in bronchitis. The juice of the fresh fruit is used in dyspepsia and as a cooling, thirst-quenching beverage in fevers and sickness.

Alkaloid in leaves = $1 - 2$, stem = 1; tannin in leaves and stem = $1 - 2$; calcium oxalate, leaves = 1; stem = $2 - 3$; fats in leaves and stem = 1; sulfur in leaves and stem = 1; peroxidase in leaves and stem = $1 - 2$.

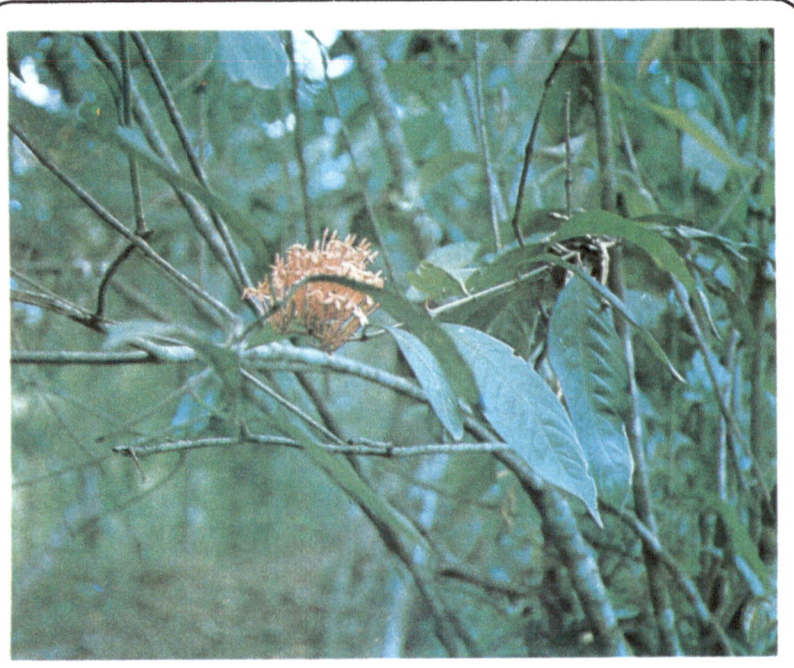

RUBIACEAE
Ixora coccinea L.
Santan-pula, santan (Tag.); *tangpupo* (Bis.).

An erect, glabrous shrub, 2 to 3 m high. Leaves sessile or subsessile, oblong, 5 to 9 cm long, base broadly cordate or rounded, apex obtuse or apiculate. Cymes, terminal, sessile or subsessile, densely many-flowered, pubescent. Calyx- teeth short, acute. Corolla pink or red, slender, the tube about 2 cm long, the lobes oblong, about 8 mm long.

Cultivated; a native of India.

Decoction of the leaves is used for sores and ulcers. Fresh stem and leaves are pounded and applied as poultice to sprains, contusion pains, eczema, furuncle and carbuncle infections. Root decoction used as a sedative in the treatment of nausea, hiccups, loss of appetite, also for irregular menstruation, amenorrhea, and cough. The root, in the form of tincture is said to be valuable remedy for diarrhea and dysentery; when diluted, it is used as gargle in sore throat. Flower decoction is a remedy for hypertension.

Saponin in leaves, stem and root = 1 − 2; tannin in leaves and stem = 2 − 3; glucosides in leaves and stem = 1; calcium oxalate, leaves and stem = 1; fats in leave and stem = 2; roots = 1; sulfur in leaves and stem = 1 − 2; peroxidase, leaves and stem and root = 2.

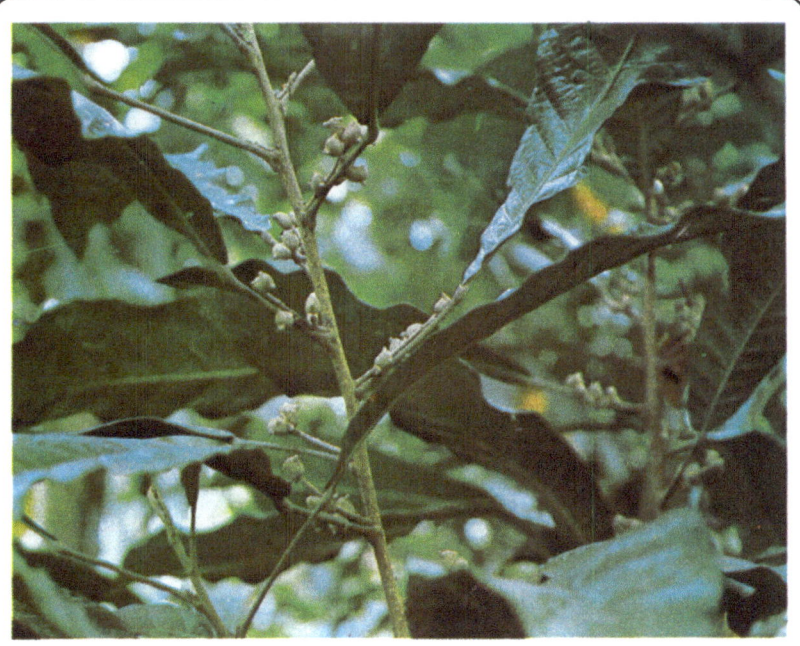

RUTACEAE
Lunasia amara Blanco
Lunas, santiki, apdong-kahoi (Tag.); *bunglai* (Bik.); *dayangdang* (Ilk.); *paitan* (Bis., Ilk.).

An erect shrub, reaching a height of 3 meters. Twigs are smooth; leaves alternately crowded obovate-oblong, 20 to 40 cm in length, and 7 to 12 cm wide, often being pointed at both ends. Male and female flowers covered with lepidote scales, small and yellow, and occur in considerable number in axillary inflorescence which are shorter than the petioles. Fruit consists of three yellowish capsules, each of which is 1 cm or more in length, is plainly marked with ribs, and opens along the veins and upper sutures.

In thickets and forests at low and medium altitudes throughout the Philippines.

Bark decoction is used for stomach troubles, and also against snake bites, together with the seeds are used to cure gastralgia in general as well as certain conditions of the digestive tract.

Alkaloids in leaves and stem = $2 - 3$; calcium oxalate, in leaves and stem = 2; formic acid, leaves and stem = 1.

43

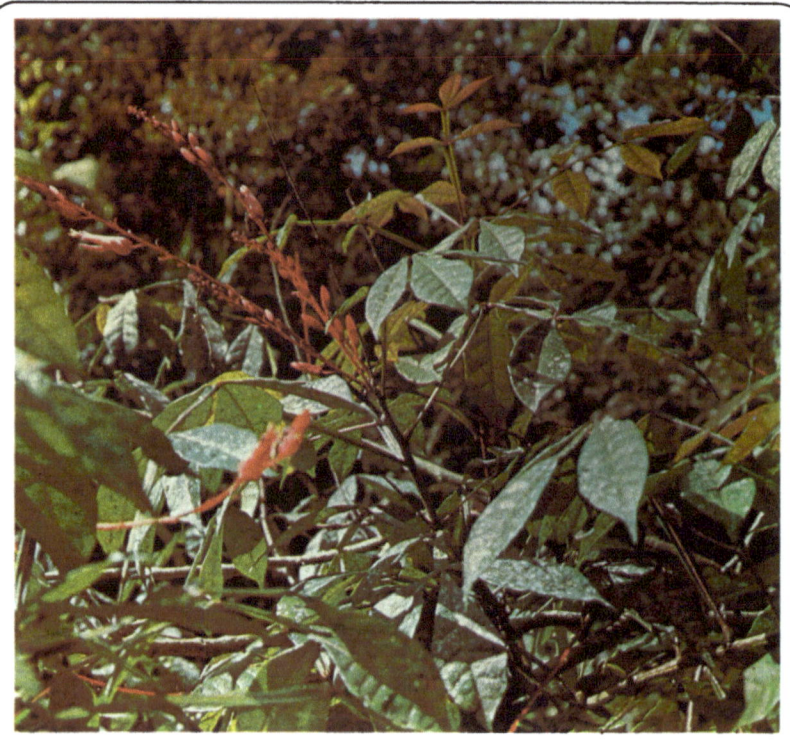

SIMARUBACEAE
Quassia amara Linn.
Corales (Sp., Tag.); *kuasia* (Tag.); bitter quassin, quassia (Engl.).

A smooth shrub growing from 2 to 3.5 m in height. The leaves alternate, about 20 cm long. Petiole and rachis are broadly winged. There are five leaflets which are stalkless and elliptic-oblong, though the terminal one may-be oblong-obovate, and 7 to 12 cm long. Flowers which are borne on racemes 8 to 20 cm long, are bright red, with the corolla about 2.5 cm long.

Cultivated for ornamental purposes.

Infusion of quassia wood is a bitter tonic, stomachic, febrifuge and anthelmintic; is given for dyspepsia, loss of appetite, debility after fever, in gout with alkaline salts, aromatics and ginger, and in dyspepsia with sulphate of zinc or iron or with mineral acids. The plant is reputed to be insecticide and is used as constituent of fly-paper.

Tannin in leaves = 2 − 3, stem = 1 − 2; calcium oxalate in leaves and roots = 1; stem = 2; sulfur in leaves = 1; fats, leaves and stem = 1; roots = 2; peroxidase in leaves = 1; stem = 2.

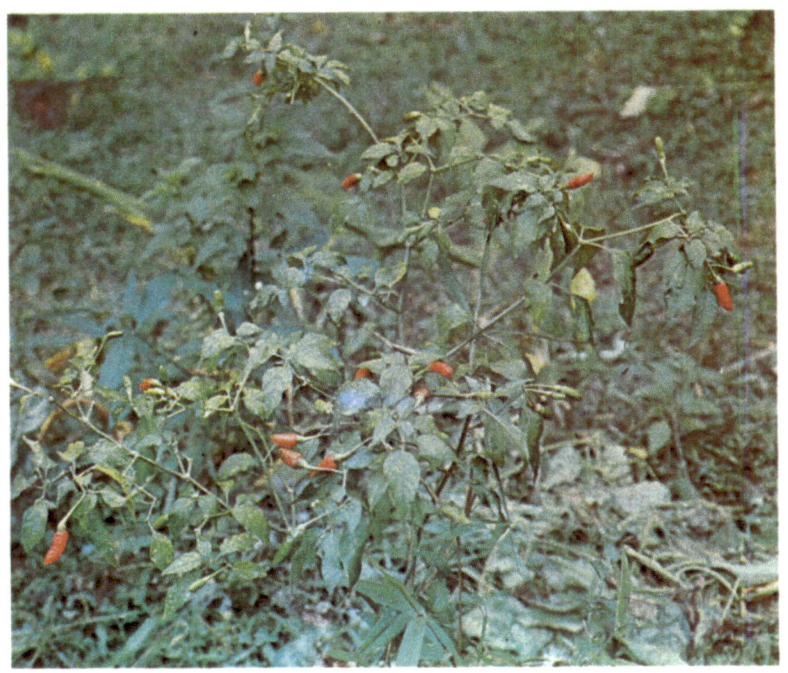

SOLANACEAE
Capsicum frutescens L.
Chili (Sp.); *pasites, sili* (Tag.); *katumbal, kitikot* (Bis.); *lagda* (Bik.); chile pepper, red pepper (Engl.).

An erect, branched, suffrutescent, shrub-like herb, 0.8 to 1.5 m high. Leaves oblong-ovate to ovate-lanceolate, acuminate, entire, 3 to 10 cm long. Flowers solitary or several in each axil, pedicelled, pale green or yellowish green, 8 to 9 mm in diameter. Fruit in the common form red, oblong-lanceolate, 1.5 to 2.5 cm long, with a very sharp taste.

In waste places, occasional, also commonly cultivated, throughout the Philippines.

Condiment, cures dyspepsia when taken moderately; externally, an irritant liniment. Sili with vinegar is an excellent stomachic; good for cholera. Externally they are strong rubefacient and act gently with no danger of vesication; they are applied as cataplasm and can be mixed with 10 to 20% of cotton seed-oil. A strong infusion of the fruit of the hotter kinds is applied as a lotion for ringworm. Ripe fruit is used as a stimulant. Warm fomentation of both leaves and fruit is applied for rheumatic pains.

Alkaloid from leaves and stems = 1 − 2; saponin in stem = 1; tannin in stem = 1; fats, leaves = 1; peroxidase, leaves = 1, stem = 2.

45

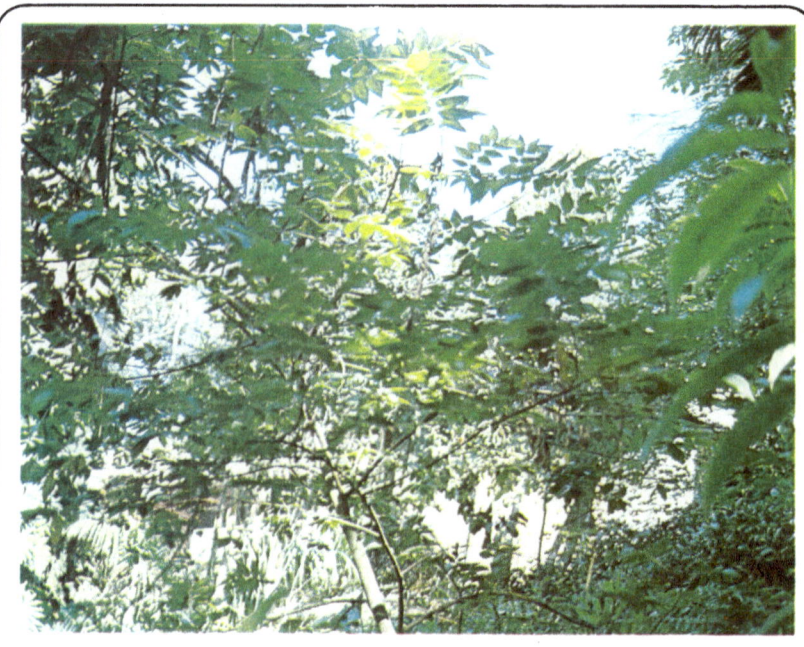

TILIACEAE
Muntingia calabura L.
Datiles, ratiles (Tag.); *cereza* (Sp.); *zanitas, seresa* (Ilk.).

A tree, 5 to 10 m high, viscid-pubescent with stellate hairs, the branches spreading. Leaves alternate, distichous, oblong, the branches oblong-lanceolate, 8 to 13 cm long, acuminate, toothed, base equilateral, one side rounded, the other acute, stipules slender, hairy, short. Flowers 2 cm in diameter, white, extra-axillary, solitary or in pairs, their pedicels erect, 1.5 to 2.5 cm long. Sepals 5, green, reflexed, lanceolate, long-acuminate, 1 cm long. Petals obovate, deciduous, 1 cm long, spreading. Stamens many. Fruit a globose, red, smooth, very fleshy, sweet berry, about 1.5 cm in diameter, filled with very numerous, small seeds.

Widely distributed in the Philippines; a native of tropical America.

Leaf decoction is antidiarrhetic. Bark decoction is used as an emollient. Infusion of the flowers is used as antispasmodic.

Datiles is very popular among Filipino children who relish its ripe fruit. From the bark a bast is obtained which is soft, pliable, and easily twisted and is used for making rope.

Saponin in leaves and stem = 2; tannin in leaves and stem = 1 − 2; fats in leaves and stem = 1; calcium oxalate, leaves and stem = 2; formic acid in leaves and stem = 2; peroxidase. leaves and stem = 1 − 2.

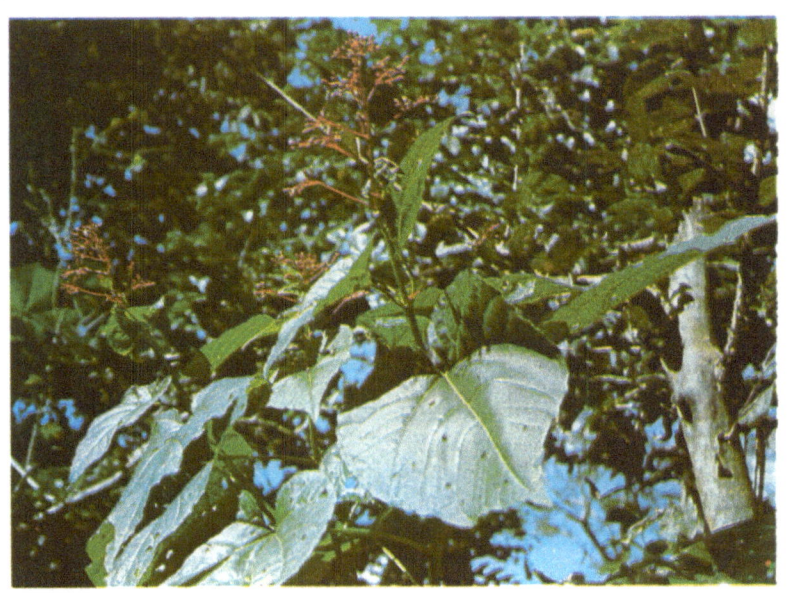

VERBENACEAE
Clerodendrum intermedium Cham.
Kasopangil (Tag.); *aloksok* (Bis.).

An erect, branched, shrubby or half-woody plant, 1 to 2 m in height. Stems are green, 4-angled. Leaves ovate being 9 to 20 cm long, with pointed tips and heart-shaped bases and shallowy toothed margins. The lower surface of the blade is covered with numerous, small but prominent glands. Flowers odorless, bright red, slender, and borne in panicles which are terminal and in the upper axils of the leaves. The corolla tube about 1 cm long, the limb spreading, somewhat oblique, subequally 5-lobed, the lobes being oblong and obtuse, 1 and 1.5 cm in diameter. The stamens are about 2 cm long, red or purplish. The fruit fleshy, blue, depressed-rounded, and about 1 cm in diameter and contains 3 to 4 seeds. The accrescent calyx red, spreading or reflexed, about 2 cm in diameter.

Found commonly in thickets, secondary forests, and open, damp places at low and medium altitude throughout the Philippines.

Leaves of this shrub are frequently used, either whole or pounded in the form of a cataplasm to relieve pains following childbirth, and for rheumatism; also used as a plaster to relieve colic in children; are applied to the abdomen of a parturient in certain complications. The young leaves are heated and while moderately warm applied on the forehead as topical in order to relieve headache. The root is known to be purgative.

Saponin in leaves = 1; fats in stem and root = 1 − 2; peroxidase in leaves, stem and root = 1 − 2; formic acid in leaves and stem = 1.

47

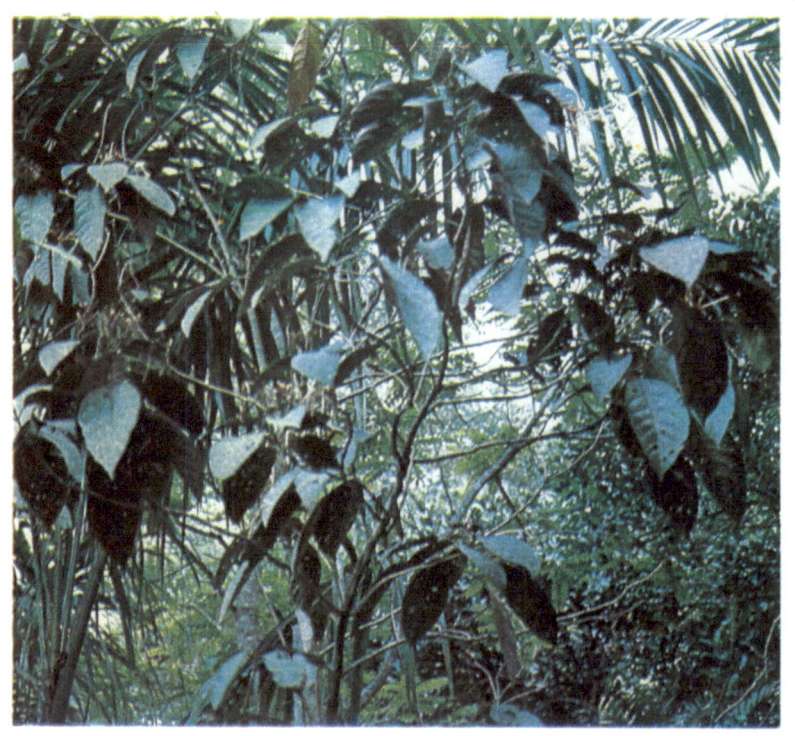

VERBENACEAE

Clerodendrum quadriloculare (Blanco) Merr.

Bagauak, bagauak-na-pula, baliktaran, salinguak (Tag.); *uak-uak* (Bis.).

An erect, glabrous or nearly glabrous shrub or small tree, 2 to 5 m high. Leaves oblong, 15 to 20 cm long, apex acuminate, base rounded, the upper surface green, the lower surface uniformly dark purple. Cymes terminal, panicled, usually many-flowered. Calyx urceolate, purple, about 1 cm long, 5-toothed. Corolla white, the tube slender, cylindric, 6 to 8 cm long, about 2 mm in diameter, the limb spreading, the lobes oblong-elliptic about 1.5 cm long. Fruit ellipsoid, 1 to 1.5 cm long, purplish, the persistent calyx red and 1 to 1.5 cm long.

Cultivated for its ornamental foliage and showy flowers. Widely distributed in forests, apparently endemic.

The leaves in topicals, are used for healing wounds and ulcers. They are also employed in tonic baths. A decoction of the leaves taken internally, and a cataplasm applied externally, are good for flatulence.

Tannin in leaves and stems = 1; glucosides in stem = 1; calcium oxalate in stem = 2; peroxidase in leaves and stem = 1; fats in leaves = 1, stem = 2.

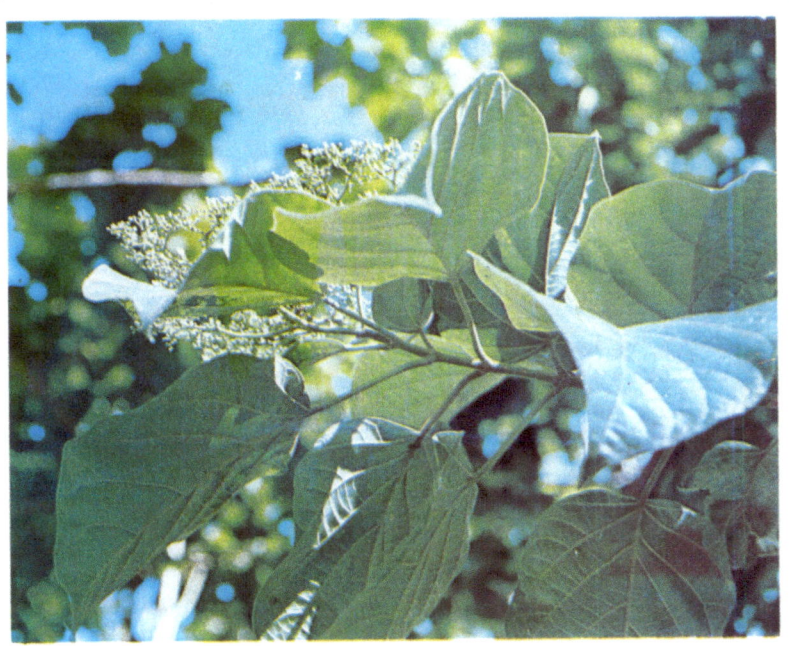

VERBENACEAE
Premna odorata Blanco
Alagaw (Tag.); *agdau* (Pang.); *anobran* (Ilk.); *pumuhat tangli* (Pamp.).

A shrub or small tree 3 to 8 m high, softly pubescent, somewhat aromatic when crushed. Leaves ovate to broadly ovate, 10 to 20 cm long, base broad, rounded or somewhat cordate, apex, acuminate, the lower surface densely pubescent. Inflorescence terminal, 8 to 20 cm in diameter. Flowers greenish white or nearly white, 4 to 5 mm long. Fruit globose, fleshy, dark purple, about 5 mm in diameter.

Common in thickets and secondary forests at a low altitude, sometimes purposely planted. Endemic.

The leaves applied over the bladder, facilitate urination; a decoction with sugar and a little "calamansi" juice taken as a drink, is effective for cough. An infusion is carminative, used for bathing babies and also as a treatment for beri-beri. A decoction of either the leaves or flowers or both is a remedy for fever caused by colds; for abdominal pains, and dysentery. Masticating the roots and swallowing the saliva is prescribed for cardiac troubles.

Alkaloids in leaves and stem = $1 - 2$; tannin in leaves and stem = $2 - 3$; glucosides in leaves and stem = 1; saponin in stem = 2.

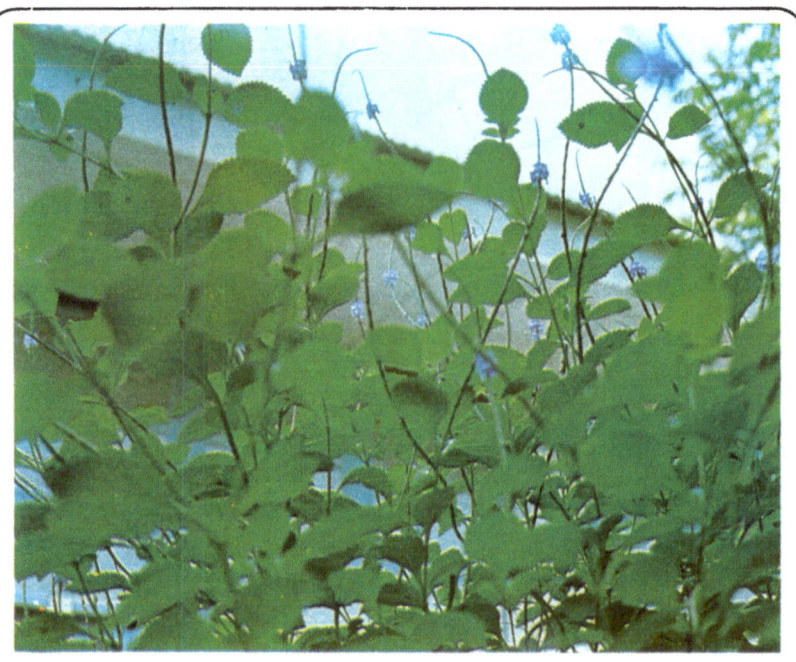

VERBENACEAE
Stachytarpheta jamaicensis (L.) Vahl
Kandi-kandilaan (Tag.); *bolo-moros* (Bik.); *albaka* (Bis.); brazilian tea, devil's coach whip (Engl.).

An erect, branched, suffrutescent herb, 1 to 15 m high, the stems terete, or the younger ones slightly angled. Leaves elliptic to oblong-ovate, acute, base decurrent on the petioles, 2.5 to 10 cm long, serrate, prominently reticulate. Corolla deep blue, about 1 cm long. Fruit enclosed in the calyx, closely appressed to and somewhat sunk in the rachis, oblong, smooth, about 4 mm long.

Common in waste places, borders of thickets, etc; throughout the Philippines.

Fresh leaves are used as topicals for ulcers; leaf decoction is given for dysentery, a cold infusion is a remedy for gonorrhea; leaf juice is used to cure eye trouble such as cataracts and for sores in children's ear; rubbed on a sprain or bruise, and as a maturative cataplasm for boils. Root decoction is abortive, and with the leaves is administered as vermifuge to children.

Saponin in leaves and stem = 1 − 2; calcium oxalate, leaves and stem = 2; fats in leaves and stem = 1; sulfur in stem = 1; formic acid in leaves = 1, stem = 2; peroxidase in stem = 1; pectic substances from leaves and stem = 2.

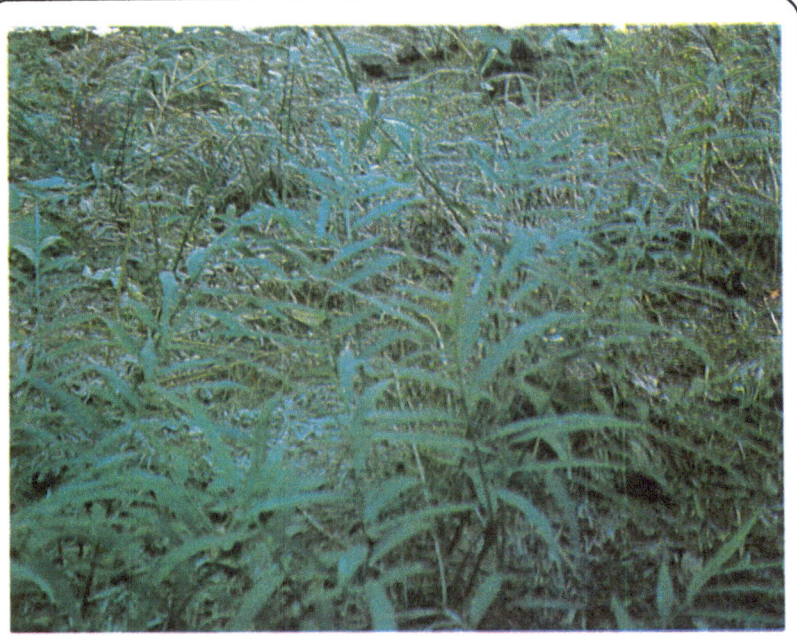

ZINGIBERACEAE
Zingiber officinale Roscoe
Luya (Tag.); *laya, baseng* (Ilk.); *agat* (Pang.); ginger (Engl.).

An erect, smooth plant rising from thickened, very aromatic rootstocks. The leafy stems, 0.4 to 1 m high. Leaves distichous, lanceolate to linear-lanceolate, 15 to 25 cm long and 2 cm wide or less. Scape erect; from the rootstocks, 15 to 25 cm high, covered with distant, imbricate bracts, the spikes ovoid to ellipsoid, dense, about 5 cm long. Bracts ovate, cuspidate, about 2.5 cm long, pale green. Calyx 1 cm long or somewhat less. Corolla greenish yellow, its tube less than 2 cm long, the lip oblong-obovate, slightly marked with purple.

Widely distributed in the Philippines in cultivation.

Pounded leaves are applied as a warm poultice to bruises. As an external medicine, the pounded rhizome alone or mixed with oil is antirheumatic and rubefacient; as a decoction, it is stomachic, stimulant, carminative and diaphoretic. Sore throat, hoarseness and loss of voice are sometimes remedied by chewing a piece of ginger. Expressed juice from fresh ginger in gradually increasing doses is a strong diuretic. Raw and crystallized ginger is used as breath sweetener, an aid to digestion, and a relief for flatulence; a cure for toothache and bleeding gums and as a strengthening agent for loose teeth and weak eyes.

Tannin in rhizomes = 1; fats in leaves and rhizomes = 2; iron in rhizomes = 1; peroxidase in rhizomes = 2; pectic substances in leaves = 2.

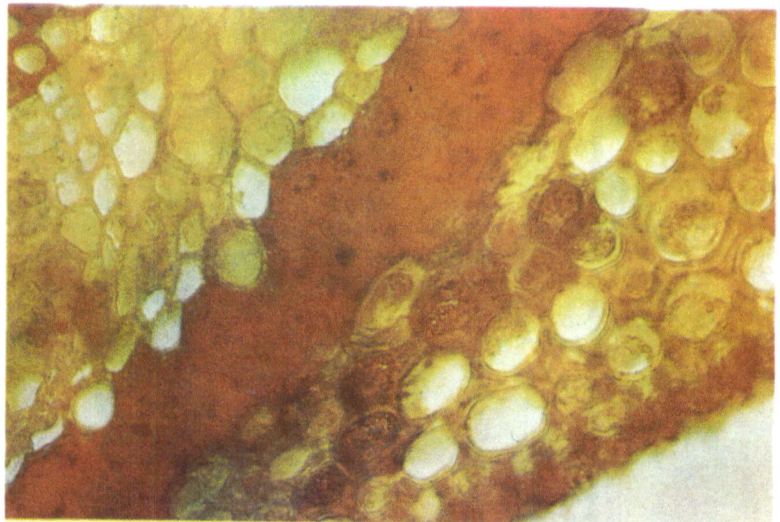

Fig. 1. Characteristic alkaloid reaction in stem section of *Clitoria ternatea.*

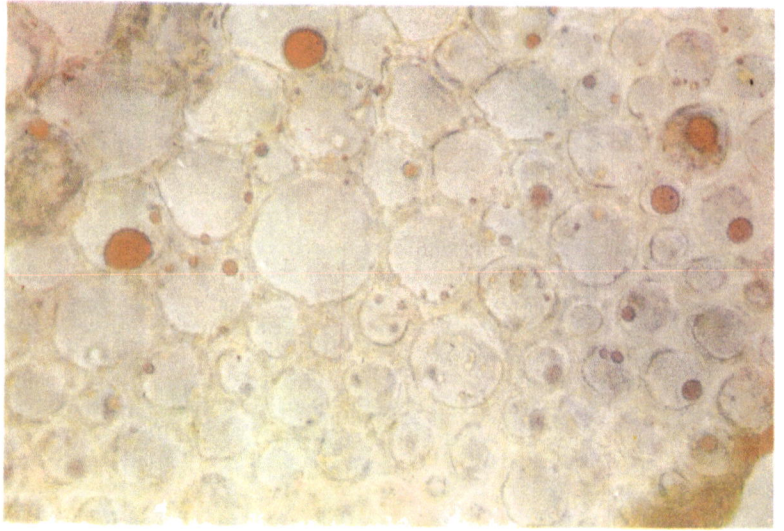

Fig. 2. Fats in *Ervatamia divaricata* leaf section.

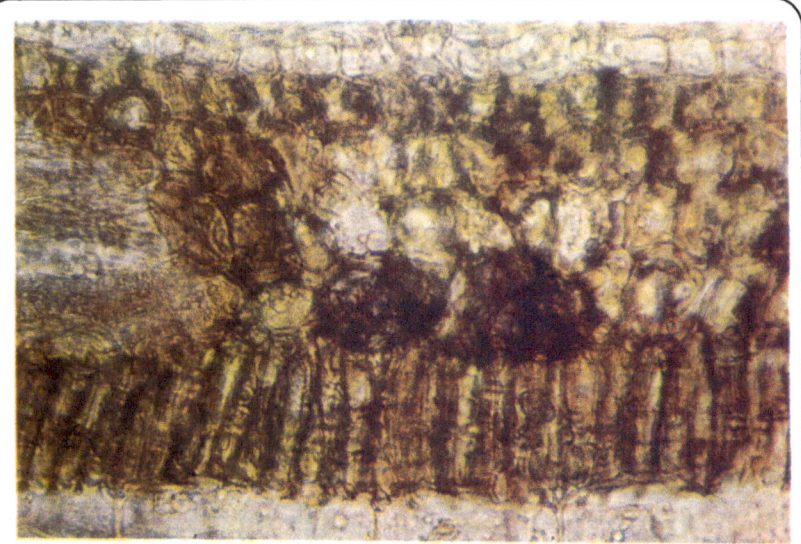

Fig. 3. Tannins in *Punica granatum* leaf section.

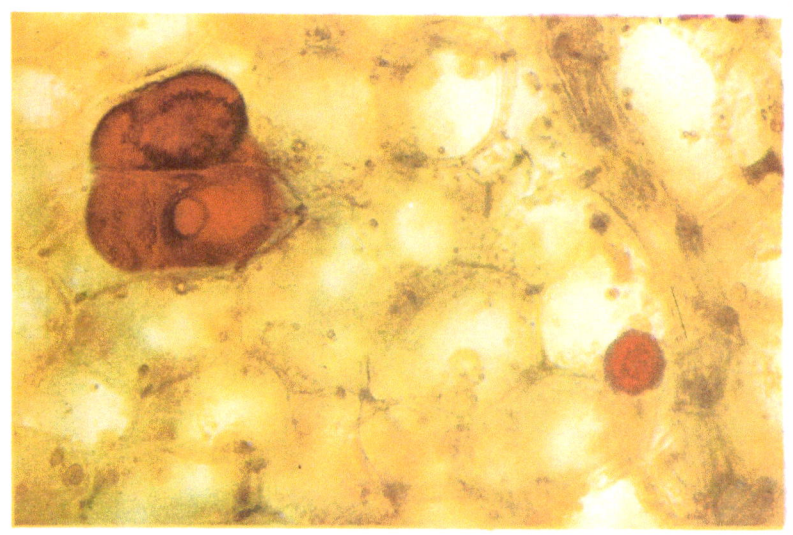

Fig. 4. Alkaloids in *Annona reticulata* stem section.

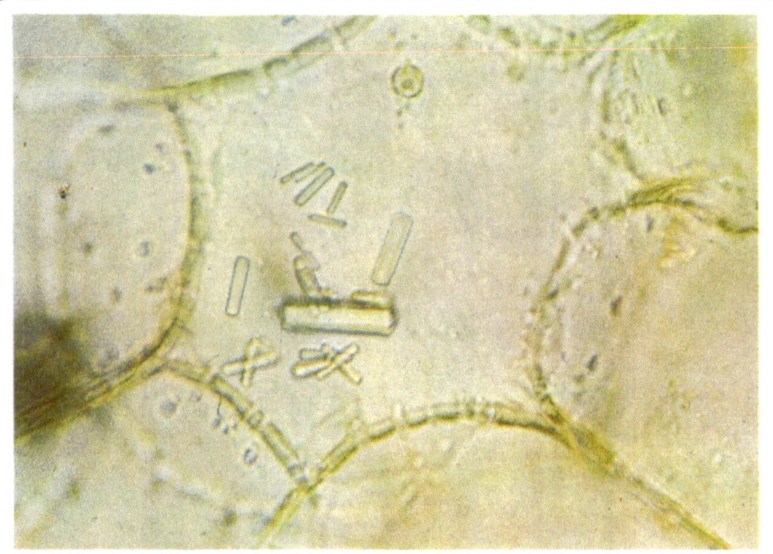

Fig. 5. Calcium oxalate crystals in *Stachytarpheta jamaicensis* stem section.

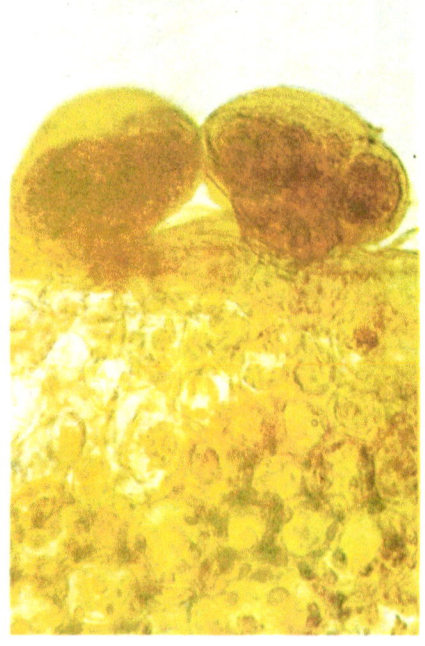

Fig. 6. Alkaloid reaction in epidermal appendages of *Gendarussa vulgaris* leaf section.

Glossary

Abortifacient – causes abortion or miscarriage.

Accrescent – enlarging with age, as with the budscales of some flowers.

Achene – a small, dry, indehiscent one-seeded fruit in which the ovary wall is free from the seed.

Active principle – the chemical component of a crude drug which has a therapeutic effect.

Acuminate – tapering to a prolonged point.

Adnate – with unlike parts congenitally grown together.

Alkaloid – a type of complex organic compound which occurs naturally in plants.

Alternative – a substance which alters a condition by a gradual change toward restoration of health.

Amenorrhea – absence of menstruation.

Analgesic – pain-reliever or pain-killer.

Anesthetic – causes total or partial loss of sensation.

Anodyne – soothing, eases pain.

Anthelmintic – expels intestinal worms.

Anticolic – relieve abdominal pain by expelling gas from the stomach and intestines.

Antidote – agents which counteract or destroy the effect of poisons or other medicines.

Antidyspeptic – acts against nausea due to indigestion.

Antiherpetic – drug for skin inflammations.

Antipyretic – substance that lowers body temperature; used against fever.

Antirheumatic – medicine for rheumatism.

Antiscorbutic – used against scurvy.

Antiseptic – an agent for destroying or inhibiting pathogenic bacteria.

Antispasmodic – prevents or relieve muscular spasms or cramps.

Antitussive – an agent that relieves coughing.

Aperients – herbs which are gently laxative.

Aperitive – stimulates bowel movement; laxative.

Aphrodisiac – stimulates sexual desire.

Areola – a small area marked out on a surface; a small pit.

Aromatic – emits fragrant odor; used to make medicinal preparations more palatable, also foods.

Arthritis – inflammation of a joint.

Astringent – shrinks tissues and prevents secretion of fluids from wounds.

Balsamic – healing or soothing agent.

Bitter tonic – stimulates salivary flow; used to increase appetite and aid digestion.

Bract – the small leaf or scale from the axil of which a flower or its pedicel proceeds.

Bulbs – modified plant buds which occur beneath the soil.

Cachexia – a condition of general ill health.

Calyx – outermost envelope of the flower, consisting of a number of sepals.

Capsule – a dry fruit of two or more carpels, dehiscent by valves.

Carbuncle – a deeply situated staphylococcal infection producing multiple adjacent draining skin sinuse (cavities or channels).

Carminative – expels gas from the alimentary canal.

Carpel – unit structure of a compound pistil.

Catarrh – inflammation of nose and mucus-membranes, with cough.

Cathartic – causes cleansing of the bowels.

Cholagogue – increases the flow of bile.

Cicatrizant – causes formation of scar tissue, healing of wounds.

Clavate – club-shaped, slender below and thickened upward.

Concoction – a preparation from crude materials, made by combining different ingredients.

Conjunctivitis – inflammation of the inner surface of the eyelid.

Contusion – injury to tissues caused by blunt force which did not disrupt or lacerate their surface; bruise.

Cordate – heart-shaped.

Coriaceous – leather-like; tough.

Corolla – petals of a flower.

Corymbose – a more or less flat-topped raceme in which the pedicels of the lower flowers are longer than those of the upper ones.

Counter-irritant – produces a blister or irritation to relieve an existing eruption elsewhere.

Crude drug – any drug, whether of vegetable or animal origin which has not undergone any chemical change but rather only some physical change such as drying and comminution.

Cuspidate – tipped with a sharp and stiff point.

Cyme – a flat or convex, open, compound flower-cluster, the inner flowers opening first.

Cystitis – infection of the urinary bladder and/or urinary tract.

Debility – weakness.

Deciduous – falling off; applied to those trees that shed all their leaves at one time.

Decoctions – solutions representing the water-soluble constituents of plant drugs prepared by boiling the drug in water.

Decongestant – tending to reduce congestion or swelling.

Decurrent – a leaf which extends in a ridge down the twig below the point of insertion.

Dehiscent – a fruit that bursts open upon maturity.

Demulcent – soothing medicine; provides a protective coating on membranes.

Deobstruent – clears obstructions of natural ducts of the body.

Depurative – purifying agent; normally applied to blood-purifiers.

Dermatitis – inflammation of the skin.

Detergent – cleansing agent.

Diaphoretic – induces excessive perspiration.

Digestive – aids digestion.

Diuretic – helps the body dispose of excess water by increasing the amount of urine produced.

Dosage form – a preparation devised to make possible the administration of medication in measured or prescribed amounts.

Dropsy – edema; excessive accumulation of fluid in body tissues.

Drupe – a fleshy fruit with a hard stone.

Dysentery – inflammation of the large intestines with evacuation of liquid, and bloody stool and tenesmus.

Dysmenorrhea – painful menstruation.

Dyspepsia – indigestion characterized by nausea.

Dysuria – difficult discharge of urine.

Ecbolic – alleviates menstrual aches and pains.

Eczema – inflammatory skin disease characterized by redness, itching and formation of scales and crusts.

Edema – abnormal accumulation of fluids in the tissues.

Elephantiasis – disease caused by infestation with a parasitic worm; characterized by the skin's becoming hard and fissured like that of an elephant's and enlargement of the affected part of the body.

Elliptic – leaf that is oval with narrowed to rounded ends.

Emetic – causes vomiting.

Emeto cathartic – causes vomiting and bowel movement.

Emmenagogue – an agent that promotes menstruation.

Emollient – softening, soothing application to the skin.

Enema – any liquid preparation introduced into the rectum.

Eupeptic – promotes good digestion.

Expectorant – promotes ejection of fluid from the lungs and trachea.

Exserted – protruded beyond, as stamens beyond the tube of the corolla.

Fascicle – a closed cluster or bundle of flowers, leaves, stems or roots.

Febrifuge – a remedy for fever.

Flatulence – gas formation in the alimentary canal.

Fluid extracts – liquid preparation of vegetable drug containing alcohol as a solvent or as a preservative or both.

Follicle – a many-seeded fruit derived from a single carpel, splitting longitudinally down one side.

Fomentation – application of warm, moist substances such as wet cloth to ease pain and inflammation.

Frutescent – shrubby.

Furuncle – local pus-forming inflammation of the skin and subcutaneous tissues.

Fusiform – spindle-shaped; tapering at each end.

Galactagogue – promotes secretion of milk.

Galenical preparations – any type of preparation, whether an extract of a crude drug or merely a solution of chemicals; pharmaceutical preparations obtained by macerating or percolating crude drugs with the appropriate menstruum carefully selected to extract as thoroughly as possible only the desired principles and to leave the inert and other undesirable principles of the plant undissolved.

Gastroenteritis – inflammation of the stomach and intestines characterized by pain, nausea and disease germs.

Germicide – destroys disease germs.

Gingivitis – inflammation of the gums.

Glabrous – smooth in the sense of having no hairs, bristles, or other pubescence.

Glaucous – having the surface covered with a waxy "bloom" or powdery material that rubs off.

Gout – a disease marked by painful inflammation of the joints.

Gum – viscous fluid exuded by some plants which discolors and hardens on exposure to air and light.

Hemorrhoid – painful swelling formed by dilatation of a vein in the anus; usually accompanied by bleeding and constipation; piles.

Herbaceous – a plant which does not develop woody tissue.

Herpes – acute skin inflammation in which clusters of small vesicles spread from one part to another.

Hirsute – with stiff or bristle hairs.

Hypnotic – induces sleep.

Imbricate – overlapping, as shingles on a roof.

Indehiscent – not opening by valves or along regular lines.
Inflorescence – the flowerhead of a plant.
Invigorant – strengthening, energy-giving agent.
Lanceolate – lance-shaped.
Latex – milky juice produced by certain plants.
Laxative – encourages defecation.
Lepidote – covered with small scales.
Liniment – a solution of an irritant drug intended to be rubbed on the skin as a counter-irritant.
Loculicidal – capsules opening by splitting through the back of each cell.
Lumbago – rheumatic pain in the lumbar region (region pertaining to the loins, part between thorax and pelvis).
Macerate – cold water extract of a plant or crude drug.
Masticatory – a substance to be chewed, but not swallowed.
Mucilage – gum-like material produced by some plants; has a soothing effect on inflamed parts.
Mumps – inflammation of the parotid glands.
Narcotic – a drug, which in moderate doses allays pain, reduces sensibility, produces sleep; in large amounts, induces stupor, coma or convulsions.
Nephritis – inflammation of the kidneys.
Nervine – soothing to the nerves; provides nervous relaxation.
Nutrient – nourishing substance.
Oblanceolate – shaped like an inverted lance.
Obovate – a flat inversely ovate body, the broad end upward.
Obovoid – shaped like an inverted egg.
Otitis media – inflammation of the middle ear.
Ovoid – a solid body ovate in outline.
Palliative – alleviates or eases a condition without curing it.
Pectoral – pertaining to the chest.
Peduncle – the stalk attached to the flower.
Pericarp – the body of the fruit developed from the ovary and enclosing the seeds.
Pharmacognosy – the study of the biology, chemistry and pharmacology of plant drugs and spices.
Pharmacology – the study of the action of chemicals and drugs in the body.
Pharyngitis – throat inflammation.
Pinna – the primary unit of a feather-like compound leaf.
Pistil – female element of a flower, consisting of stigma, style and ovary.
Poultice – a soft, usually heated preparation spread on a cloth applied to a sore or inflammation.
Prophylactic – preventing against disease.
Prostrate – trailing on the ground.
Pubescent – hairy or downy, especially with fine and soft hairs or pubescence.
Pulmonary – pertaining to the lungs.
Purgative – causing evacuation from the intestines.
Pyorrhea – discharge of pus from gums.
Pyrosis – a stomach disorder characterized by burning sensation with eructations of acid fluids.
Raceme – a simple inflorescence in which the elongated axis bears a number of flowers with short stems of nearly equal length.
Rachis – the axis of an inflorescence or other body.
Reactivator – restores to a state of activity.

Receptacle — generally enlarged end of flower stalk.
Refrigerant — relieving fever and thirst.
Rejuvenator — causes renewed vitality.
Restorative — aids in regaining normal vigor.
Revulsive — diverts disease from one part of the body to another.
Rhizome — an underground stem.
Rubefacient — an external skin application causing redness of the skin.
Saponin — a plant glycoside which foams in water.
Scabrid — somewhat rough.
Scandent — climbing.
Scape — a peduncle rising from the ground or near it, and bearing one or
    more flowers.
Sedative — calms the nerves.
Sepal — a segment of calyx.
Seriate — arranged in a series of rows.
Serrulate — finely saw-toothed.
Sessile — without a stalk of any kind.
Setaceous — bristle like.
Soporific — induces sleep.
Spathe — a bract which encloses an inflorescence.
Specific — agent or remedy that has a special effect on a particular disease.
Spike — elongated inflorescence with sessile or nearly-sessile flowers.
Stamens — the male organs of the flower.
Stimulant — increases or hastens body activity.
Stomachic — stimulates activity of the stomach.
Stomatitis — inflammation of the mouth.
Styptic — stops bleeding with an astringent.
Succulent — leaf texture which is soft and fleshy, usually thick.
Sudorific — inducing sweat; diaphoretic.
Suffrutescent — slightly shrubby or woody.
Sulcate — grooved with deep furrows.
Suppuration — pus formation.
Taeniafuge — expels tapeworm.
Tannins — a group of astringent plant constituents.
Tenesmus — the sensation of a need to evacuate the bladder or bowels with-
    out result.
Therapeutics — branch of medicine associated with the use of remedies and
    the treatment of diseases.
Tincture — alcoholic extract of a plant drug.
Tonic — produces healthy muscular condition and reaction.
Truncate — as if cut off at the top.
Tuber — a swollen underground stem.
Tympanitis — inflammation of the middle ear.
Ulcer — a superficial inflammation or sore of the skin or mucus membrane
    discharging pus.
Umbel — an umbrella-shaped inflorescence.
Vermicide — kills worms.
Vermifuge — expels worms.
Vesicant — a blistering application.
Vulnerary — used in the healing of wounds.
Whorl — three or more structures at a node, as leaves, branches or floral parts.

Index

Piper betle	40
Punica granatum	41
Quassia amara	45
Premna odorata	49

Antiseptic
Manihot esculenta	14
Streblus asper	33
Piper betle	40

Antitussive and Antiasthmatic
Gendarussa vulgaris	3
Mangifera indica	5
Ervatamia divaricata	7
Bixa orellana	9
Ceiba pentandra	10
Quisqualis indica	12
Phyllanthus reticulatus	15
Ocimum sanctum	17
Cajanus cajan	21
Cassia occidentalis	22
Clitorea ternatea	24
Sesbania grandiflora	26
Tamarindus indica	28
Hibiscus rosa sinensis	29
Moringa oleifera	34
Jasminum sambac	37
Averrhoa bilimbi	38
Averrhoa carambola	39
Punica granatum	41
Ixora coccinea	42
Premna odorata	49

Aphrodisiac
Ceiba pentandra	10
Artocarpus heterophyllus	32
Piper betle	40

Astringent
Mangifera indica	5
Ceiba pentandra	10
Kalanchoe pinnata	13
Phyllanthus reticulatus	15
Streblus asper	33

Carminative
Pogostemon cablin	18
Syzygium cuminiii	35
Piper betle	40
Lunasia amara	43
Capsicum frutescens	44
Premna odorata	51
Zingiber officinale	51

Moringa oleifera	34
Syzygium cuminii	35
Mirabilis jalapa	36
Premna odorata	49
Zingiber officinale	51

For Earache
Graptophyllum pictum	2
Gendarussa vulgaris	3
Kalanchoe pinnata	13
Ocimum sanctum	17
Clitorea ternatea	24
Stachytarpheta jamaicensis	50

Emmenagogue
Graptophyllum pictum	2
Gendarussa vulgaris	3
Impatiens balsamina	8
Pogostemon cablin	18
Hibiscus rosa sinensis	29
Averrhoa carambola	39
Ixora coccinea	42

For Eye trouble
Ervatamia divaricata	7
Kalanchoe pinnata	13
Phyllanthus reticulatus	15
Coleus scutellarioides	16
Caesalpinia pulcherrima	20
Tamarindus indica	28
Hibiscus rosa sinensis	29
Jasminum sambac	37
Stachytarpheta jamaicensis	50

Galactagogue
Amaranthus spinosus	4
Moringa oleifera	34
Averrhoa carambola	39

For Gonorrhea
Ocimum sanctum	17
Cassia occidentalis	22
Hibiscus rosa sinensis	29
Stachytarpheta jamaicensis	50

For Headache
Quisqualis indica	12
Manihot esculenta	14
Coleus scutellarioides	16
Persea americana	19
Piliostigma malabarica	23
Sesbania grandiflora	26
Averrhoa carambola	39
Clerodendrum intermedium	47

For Skin diseases, boils and abscesses
- *Amaranthus spinosus* — 4
- *Mangifera indica* — 5
- *Ervatamia divaricata* — 7
- *Impatiens balsamina* — 8
- *Bixa orellana* — 9
- *Durio zibethenius* — 11
- *Quisqualis indica* — 12
- *Kalanchoe pinnata* — 13
- *Manihot esculenta* — 14
- *Ocimum sanctum* — 17
- *Cassia occidentalis* — 22
- *Gliricidia sepium* — 25
- *Syzygium cuminii* — 35
- *Mirabilis jalapa* — 36
- *Ixora coccinea* — 42
- *Capsium frutescens* — 44

For Snakebites and insect bites
- *Impatiens balsamina* — 8
- *Kalanchoe pinnata* — 13
- *Artocarpus heterophyllus* — 32
- *Streblus asper* — 33
- *Moringa oleifera* — 34
- *Lunasia amara* — 43

Tonic
- *Durio zibethenius* — 11
- *Caesalpinia pulcherrima* — 20
- *Cassia occidentalis* — 22
- *Quassia amara* — 45
- *Clerodendrum quadriloculare* — 48

For Toothache
- *Ervatamia divaricata* — 7
- *Kalanchoe pinnata* — 13
- *Persea americana* — 19

Vulnerary
- *Graptophyllum pictum* — 2
- *Ervatamia divaricata* — 7
- *Manihot esculenta* — 14
- *Coleus scutellarioides* — 16
- *Cajanus cajan* — 21
- *Pithecellobium dulce* — 27
- *Tamarindus indica* — 28
- *Artocarpus heterophyllus* — 32
- *Streblus asper* — 33
- *Syzygium cuminii* — 34
- *Jasminum sambac* — 37
- *Ixora coccinea* — 42
- *Clerodendrum quadriloculare* — 48
- *Stachytarpheta jamaicensis* — 50

Bibliography

Brown, W. H. 1941. Useful Plants of the Philippines. Manila. Bureau of Printing.

Claus, E. P., V. E. Taylor and C. R. Brady. 1970. Pharmacognosy. Lea and Febiger. Philadelphia.

Co, L. L. 1977. A Manual on Some Philippine Medicinal Plants. Diliman, Quezon City.

Coon, Nelson. 1963. Using Plants for Healing. Hearthside Press, Inc. New York.

Ferguson, N. M. 1956. A Textbook of Pharmacognosy. New York. MacMillan and Co.

Githens, T. S. 1948. Drug Plants of Africa. University of Pennsylvania.

Grieve, M. .959. A Modern Herbal. New York. Hafner Publishing Company.

Johansen, D. A. 1940. Plant Microtechnique. New York. John Wiley and Sons, Inc.

Lehner, Ernst and Johanna. 1962. Folklore and Odysseys of Food and Medicinal Plants. New York. Tudor Publishing Co.

Lucas, R. Nature's Medicines. London. Neville. Spearman.

Lugod, G. C. and J. V. Pancho. Undated. Medicinal Plants of the College of Agriculture Arboretum and Vicinity.

Merrill, E. D. 1912. A Flora of Manila. Manila Bureau of Printing.

Nelson, A. 1951. Medical Botany. Edinburgh. E. S. Livingstone Ltd.

Quisumbing, E. 1951. Medicinal Plants of the Philippines. Manila. Bureau of Printing.

Trease, G. E. and W. C. Evans. 1972. Pharmacognosy. London, Balliere-Tindall.

Sulit, M. D. 1947. Local medicinal plants sold in the City of Manila. v.1/Department of Agriculture and Commerce Bulletin.

Sulit, M. D. 1958. Medicinal Plants used by ethnic groups of the Philippines: their preparation and application. Jour. Phil. Phar. Assoc.

Taylor, N. 1965. Plant drugs that changed the world. New York. Dodd, Mead and Co.

Uphof, J. C. Th. 1959. Dictionary of economic plants. New York. Hafner Publishing Company.

Valenzuela, P., J. A. Concha and A. C. Santos. 1949. Constituents, Uses and Pharmacopoeia of Some Philippine Medicinal Plants. The Phil. Jour. of Forestry. v.6. Bureau of Printing.